A Professional's Guide to Small-Group Personal Training

Keli Roberts

ACSM-EP, ACE Gold PT, GFI, HC, AFAA

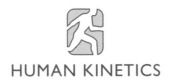

HUMAN KINETICS

Library of Congress Cataloging-in-Publication Data

Names: Roberts, Keli, 1961- author.
Title: A professional's guide to small group personal training / Keli
  Roberts.
Description: Champaign, IL : Human Kinetics, [2022] | Includes
  bibliographical references and index.
Identifiers: LCCN 2020025872 (print) | LCCN 2020025873 (ebook) | ISBN
  9781492546801 (paperback) | ISBN 9781492546818 (pdf) | ISBN
  9781718201187 (epub)
Subjects: LCSH: Personal trainers--Training of. | Personal
  trainers--Vocational guidance. | Physical education and training--Study
  and teaching. | Small groups.
Classification: LCC GV428.7 .R63 2022 (print) | LCC GV428.7 (ebook) | DDC
  613.7/1023--dc23
LC record available at https://lccn.loc.gov/2020025872
LC ebook record available at https://lccn.loc.gov/2020025873

Acquisitions Editor: Diana Vincer; **Developmental Editor:** Laura Pulliam; **Managing Editor:** Miranda K. Baur; **Copyeditor:** Heather Gauen Hutches; **Indexer:** Andrea Hepner; **Permissions Manager:** Dalene Reeder; **Graphic Designer:** Denise Lowry; **Cover Designer:** Keri Evans; **Cover Design Specialist:** Susan Rothermel Allen; **Photograph (cover):** Ridofranz/iStock/Getty Images; **Photographs (interior):** Graham Koffler/© Human Kinetics, unless otherwise noted; **Photo Asset Manager:** Laura Fitch; **Photo Production Specialist:** Amy M. Rose; **Photo Production Manager:** Jason Allen; **Senior Art Manager:** Kelly Hendren; **Illustrations:** © Human Kinetics, unless otherwise noted; **Printer:** Sheridan Books

We thank Breakthru Fitness in Pasadena, California, for assistance in providing the location for the photo shoot for this book.

Human Kinetics books are available at special discounts for bulk purchase. Special editions or book excerpts can also be created to specification. For details, contact the Special Sales Manager at Human Kinetics.

Printed in the United States of America   10 9 8 7 6 5 4 3 2 1

The paper in this book is certified under a sustainable forestry program.

Human Kinetics
1607 N. Market Street
Champaign, IL 61820
USA

United States and International
Website: **US.HumanKinetics.com**
Email: info@hkusa.com
Phone: 1-800-747-4457

Canada
Website: **Canada.HumanKinetics.com**
Email: info@hkcanada.com

E7020

Tell us what you think!
Human Kinetics would love to hear what we can do to improve the customer experience. Use this QR code to take our brief survey.

I dedicate this book to my family and loved ones. My mother encouraged me to read; it gave me a passion and appreciation for writing. My father birthed my love of all things active and competitive. My brothers, Ricky, Steven, and Byron, taught me what it was to be tough and resilient. I appreciate my stepfather, Joey, for always believing in me. And I thank my partner, Greg, for the unconditional love and support.

CONTENTS

PREFACE

Growing up in Brisbane, Australia, in the 1960s and '70s, I started competitively swimming when I was five years old, and I continued to love and excel in all sports throughout my school years. After graduating, I went on to work as a model in Sydney, then in Italy, Switzerland, Germany, and France. After living in Europe for two years, I came back to Australia, disenchanted with the fashion industry, and quit modeling. In an effort to get healthy and lose some weight, I rediscovered sports and fitness—and most significantly, aerobics! I fell in love with aerobics! In 1986, I took a course through the organization ACHPER (now known as the Australian Institute of Fitness) and became a registered Fitness Leader. I had found my mission in life: to make a difference in people's lives through health and fitness.

Back in the mid-1980s when I got certified, very few instructors had any sort of teaching credential. Most group fitness leaders got their start when the scheduled teacher didn't show up, and they got pulled to the front of the class, where they would do a lot of kicks and knee lifts. I saw a need! It was obvious to me that more instructors needed to be certified and that further education was vital.

In 1988, I met Lynn Brick, a master instructor who had come to Sydney to do workshops for a club I was teaching at. At the same time, I bought a copy of the IDEA Foundation group fitness instructor manual and started studying it. The path became clear: I knew I needed to continue my education. I wanted to get a hands-on education, so I saved my money and flew to Los Angeles.

When I arrived in Los Angeles in 1990, all I wanted to do was learn. I came to take the IDEA Foundation exam (now ACE) and took classes from the best of the best at Voight Fitness and Dance in West Hollywood. Little did I know then that my career would take off in the direction that it did, but it has been a dream come true. In 1991, I started my own personal training business and was also chosen to lead a step workout video with Cher (a singer and actress whose work has earned her a Grammy, Emmy, Golden Globe, and Academy Award). The video sold so well and received such positive feedback that I signed a contract to develop and teach a video series of my own through CBS/Fox. Known as the "Trainer to the Stars" in the early '90s, with a prestigious clientele of Hollywood celebrities, my career in the fitness industry was launched in the consumer market through the media work I did to promote Cher's *A New Attitude* video and my own Real Fitness series. It was an exciting time. I found myself flying around the world to promote videos while touring with Cher as her personal trainer—while I was just starting my PT business.

I was yet to achieve my dreams of teaching continuing education, but I knew that was what I wanted. During the early to mid-'90s I established myself as a continuing education presenter; as my opportunities grew, I started earning recognition. I have since presented at conferences around the world, including in Israel, Brazil, England, Scotland, Ireland, Germany, Italy, France, Spain, Portugal, Japan, China, Thailand, Belgium, and Canada.

With every convention I taught at and each country I visited, I continued to learn valuable teaching tools—whether it was from teaching in a foreign language, presenting with a translator, or simply having my nonverbal teaching skills to rely on. These experiences brought me to where I am today, hoping that my lessons can be passed on to the readers of this book.

Whether you're just starting out as a trainer or you've had a training business for a while and want to branch out into the world of small-group training (SGT), *A Professional's Guide to Small-Group Personal Training* will be a comprehensive step-by-step copilot on this exciting fitness journey. My hope is that this guide will provide answers that are not available elsewhere. Whether that's a business concern or safety-related query or something in the realm of teaching, coaching, and communication, this book has something for everyone.

From chapter 1, you'll find out the opportunities that this type of business provides and learn what it takes to be successful. Chapter 2 offers information on the practice of keeping your business secure. Chapter 3 guides you through creating a plan for building your dream business. As the saying goes, if you fail to plan, you plan to fail! If you're opening a small studio or own a gym and are looking for ideas, the In the Trenches sections offer inspiration and ideas on how to set up your business. In chapter 4, you'll learn to build your client base with easy-to-implement tools for retention and referrals as well as tips and ideas to help you market your SGT business.

One of the primary differences between traditional group fitness classes and SGT classes (other than class numbers) is in assessment and exercise testing services provided. Chapter 5 is filled with protocols for a variety of assessments and exercise tests you'll find indispensable. By offering these essential services to your clients, you'll add real value to your sessions. To better understand your clients, in chapter 6, you'll review the transtheoretical model of behavioral change, examine skill development, and learn some essential tools to foster your multilevel teaching skills. Then, in chapter 7, you'll further refine your communication by incorporating the different ways that people learn—verbally, visually, and kinesthetically—and you will acquire some indispensable verbal coaching techniques. Chapter 8 offers essential strategies to optimize group achievement to help you motivate and engage your groups. Chapter 9 covers the programming components and training variables, providing you with an in-depth review of the principles of exercise program design. The real fun begins in chapter 10 with an in-depth look at advanced training techniques and modalities. You'll examine recent HIIT-based research and see how this can be applied in an SGT setting.

No workout program is complete without an effective warm-up and cool-down; chapter 11 provides you with ideas and strategies designed to keep your groups safe. Various stretching modalities are examined, offering you the up-to-date information you'll need to choose what's best for your classes.

Knowing how to work with all fitness levels is essential but not always easy. From the chapter 12 introductory training programs, you'll take away three different programs, including a workout to enhance posture using simple equipment such as resistance bands, stability balls, and suspension training systems. The easy-to-replicate workouts in this chapter will accommodate your less-conditioned groups, helping them get off to the right start.

The six advanced training programs you'll find in chapter 13 are fun and will present a genuine progressive challenge to your class participants. Each program caters to well-conditioned individuals looking to take their fitness to the next level. Some of these programs incorporate specialized equipment such as rowers, BOSU balls, and ropes. If you don't have access to these, you can use the concept of the program and make it your own with the equipment you have. All the workouts will allow customization to provide your clients with the most suitable exercise programs. Feel free to substitute movements that work best for your groups.

One of the great advantages that an SGT setting offers is the camaraderie that working in small groups offers. Chapter 14 provides you with team-building workouts that incorporate partner training, team training, and more. The kettlebells, medicine balls, suspension training systems, resistance bands, and other small devices used in these programs make them affordable to implement.

Finally, you'll find selected exercises, with photos and descriptions, in chapter 15. This final chapter covers the more unusual and unique exercises you may not be familiar with.

My hope is that you'll find this book helpful and that you'll use this step-by-step process to construct the SGT business of your dreams.

ACKNOWLEDGMENTS

I'd like to acknowledge the following people for helping me on my journey:

- Dr. Len Kravitz, for all your brilliant research and your ability to make complex information easy to understand.

- Fabio Comana, MS; Douglas Brooks, MS; Candice Brooks; and Jay Blahnik, for your contribution to my education as a trainer and instructor.

- Sara Kooperman, JD, for your faith in me as an educator and faculty member for SCW Fitness Education.

- Henry Segal, for giving me my first job in the United States; you launched my career here!

- Laura Pulliam, my ever-patient and encouraging editor: I don't know how you do it! You have an amazing knack, and there's no way I could've done this without you.

- Michelle and Phil Dozois at Breakthru Fitness in Pasadena: I'm beyond grateful that you provided me with such an incredible space for the shoot. And a special thanks to the team of trainers at Breakthru that inspired several of the advanced programs featured in the book.

- My fantastic team of models who worked so hard for the photo shoot (Eric Thompson, Heidi Hoff, Nicole Fahnestock, Toby Massenburg, Camden Crane, and Jason Dalcour): Thank you, I couldn't have done this without you! I am truly blessed.

- The American Council on Exercise, for helping me learn my craft as a personal trainer, group fitness instructor, and health coach and for having confidence in me as a master trainer presenting live courses.

- The American College of Sports Medicine, for the in-depth education and the many opportunities to present at the International Health and Fitness Summit.

- My personal training clients: Your loyalty and hard work deserve many thanks.

- The participants who take my classes: You've taught me so much; I'm beyond grateful.

- The instructors who participate in my continuing education presentations and certifications: You've allowed me the opportunity to live my dream.

- My fellow educators and the presenters who've worked with me throughout my career: Thank you for your wisdom and friendship.

PART I

THE BUSINESS OF SMALL-GROUP PERSONAL TRAINING

CHAPTER 1

Understanding Small-Group Personal Training

Group fitness training first gained popularity in the late 1960s and early 1970s, when Dr. Kenneth Cooper revolutionized the concept of fitness by coining the word *aerobics*. Innovative dance instructors such as Jacki Sorensen, Judi Sheppard Missett, Richard Simmons, and Jane Fonda created easy-to-follow dance exercises that became the first intentional group exercise classes, setting the framework for the future of group fitness programs.

Group fitness has since experienced a vast evolution, going beyond aerobics to attract a much wider audience. With a greater emphasis on goal-directed specializations, participants can now choose from classes as varied as indoor rowing, indoor cycling, circuit training, strength training, and more. Many group training classes have progressed to a more scientific approach, with an emphasis on functional movement. Workouts are now designed to make performance of everyday activity easier, smoother, safer, and more efficient, with the main goal of improving the participants' quality of life (Yoke & Kennedy, 2003).

As a result of the expanded concept of group fitness, teaching methods have also evolved from having participants simply watch and mimic to a more personalized and inclusive experience. Much of this evolution has been influenced not just by the group fitness training world, but also by personal training. A customized, personal workout designed by a qualified professional around the client's needs, goals, and priorities is ideal for many gym-goers—except for the price point. Personal training's appeal can fade when costs are a consideration. For most health clubs, members pay a monthly fee, and if they want to add a personal trainer, the additional costs can be significant. However, traditional group exercise is typically included as part of a gym membership.

Group training can help people commit to regular physical activity. According to one study of 3,806 urban adult New Yorkers, men and women who were physically active as part of a group or with a partner reported 1.4 times more activity than those who exercise alone (Firestone, Yi, Bartley, & Eisenhower,

2015). Other researchers have also found that social support is a key factor in a person's decision to perform a healthy behavior. Many participants enjoy the energy, teamwork, camaraderie, and friendly competition of being in a group, but they would also prefer a more personalized experience. These clients want focused attention from the instructor as well as the community feel of group training. That's where small-group training comes in.

What Is Small-Group Training?

Small-group training (SGT) is a hybrid of group exercise and personal training. In small-group training, the feedback is more specific and individualized, similar to one-on-one settings, while incorporating the energy and teamwork of traditional group exercise.

Small-group training first debuted on the Top 20 Fitness Trends list of the American College of Sports Medicine (ACSM) in 2007 (Thompson, 2006) and has continued as a major trend for the past decade. According to ACSM, a certified personal trainer (CPT) must be creative in the way they package personal training sessions due to clients' decreasing personal income and discretionary spending. Training a small group of two to six people makes good economic sense for both the trainer and the client. The 2017 ACSM Annual Survey of Fitness Trends (Thompson, 2016) also includes many trends that can potentially be combined for a cutting-edge program—for example, using wearable technology while doing bodyweight HIIT that includes strength and functional training for weight loss.

What Are the Attributes of Small-Group Training Instructors?

Group fitness instructors (GFIs) and certified personal trainers (CPTs) have similar foundational education in exercise physiology and human movement, which provides them with base knowledge in training. There are a couple of differences; GFIs often have great charisma and group motivational skills, whereas CPTs have experience in designing specific programs and developing rapport with their clients. When these talents are combined, trainers can provide a successful and motivating experience that is personalized for their participants needs and goals. This is the art of SGT instruction: the combination of providing a personalized program with masterful presentation skills.

To be successful, a small-group training instructor needs certain personality attributes. Enthusiasm, passion, and charisma go a long way. Although anyone with a basic knowledge of training can learn how to write a program, not everyone can motivate groups. Being creative, spontaneous, and energetic, with a passion for making a difference in people's lives, elevates great training to an exceptional experience. Consider how your own personal style can drive your small-group training business.

Although it might not seem so, the personal relationship between an SGT instructor and their client is important. The relationship begins from the first meeting, whether over the phone, through email, or in person. Being professional, organized, and knowledgeable builds trust; being creative, spontaneous, and energetic maintains the client's interest and motivation. Communicating masterfully, having compassion, and being positive, genuine, and kind builds relationships. All these elements together shape the relationships you have with your groups.

The following personality attributes are important for a successful SGT instructor to have:

- *Enthusiasm.* Enthusiasm helps create a motivating environment when working with groups.
- *Professionalism.* Professionalism can be as simple as being punctual and reliable, as well as having consistent services available for billing.
- *Expertise.* With the fitness industry constantly changing and growing, having a solid foundation of knowledge and staying updated is essential.
- *Creativity.* Being creative is more than simply coming up with new exercises or programs. It can also involve creative problem solving through excellent communication skills.
- *Spontaneity.* It's always good to be able to think on your feet: Equipment, weather, and number of participants are all things that can change fast. Having a plan B and being able to spontaneously change course is an art.
- *Compassion.* People don't care about how much you know until they know how much you care. Having a caring personality helps build stronger relationships.
- *Communication.* As an instructor, one of your primary skills should be your ability to communicate effectively as well as listen actively.
- *Motivation.* It's impossible to motivate others if you're not motivated yourself. Find what motivates you and work from there.
- *Energy.* As a trainer, your energy is your currency. Your business relies on it.
- *Organization.* To succeed in the fitness business, it takes more than knowledge and a fit-looking body—being organized is also part of your professional responsibility.
- *Positivity.* Staying positive will help your groups stay focused and engaged.
- *Sincerity.* Empathy, warmth, and genuineness are all essential in the development of rapport and strong relationships.
- *Passion.* Training can often involve long hours of hard work, but your passion will drive you forward.
- *Charisma.* When working with groups, charisma can set you apart from your competition. It's a mixture of passion, energy, having a positive outlook, being motivated, and having a true purpose for what you do.

What Are the Settings for Small-Group Training?

There are many different settings in which an SGT instructor can work, from exclusive boutique studios to big commercial multipurpose clubs. It is important to consider whether you want to run your own business or be an employee, as well as what populations you want to train, the space available, and your specializations and goals. Working for someone can provide job security, many potential clients, a training location, and health and retirement benefits. Having your own business allows you more freedom, but at the cost of having to find your own clients, which can be a considerable challenge. Furthermore, you must pay expenses such as rent, equipment, and business owner policy insurance.

Commercial fitness clubs such as Orange Theory (USA) offer small-group personal training with classes of 5 to 10 people, and CrossFit boxes accommodate 5 to 15 people per group. The commonality of these businesses is that they offer a more personalized, goal-driven approach to group training. Small-group Pilates is also extremely popular, again providing participants with a personalized approach to fitness with the motivation benefits of group training.

Corporate wellness and fitness is an area that has grown in the past several years, with many large companies investing in disease prevention. It's not uncommon for large corporations to have sophisticated training facilities available to employees. This is a huge opportunity for trainers. It's worth investigating banking and investment, entertainment, manufacturing, and retail companies to see if they're interested in offering small-group fitness training for their employees. Many will welcome the team-building experience of group training.

Sports-specific training groups are another great option. Golf, for example, is often played by people who have time and expendable income and are frequently willing to spend what it takes to improve. Tennis players often look for off-court programs to enhance on-court performance as well. Country clubs also frequently offer tennis or golf training to their members, leading to opportunities for trainers who have a good working knowledge of these sports. If you're interested in these sports, this can be a particularly enjoyable opportunity.

Triathlon is another fast-growing sport whose athletes greatly benefit from conditioning to improve strength and flexibility, especially in the off-season. During the winter months, you might offer an injury prevention class that concentrates on building balance for the typically under- and overused muscles. Check with your local running, swimming, and triathlon clubs for opportunities. Renting space in a studio or even meeting in a park can provide the setting for your group.

Boot camp–style classes also fall into the category of small-group training and are often taught outdoors, including in parks or even on beaches. Participants enjoy the energy of the group and the goal-specific focus as well as the outdoor setting. Barry's Bootcamp, a small-group treadmill and weight-training format that originated in 1998, is an example of a successful business derived from traditional military-inspired boot camp classes. Tabata Bootcamp, another small-group training program, is taught using a high-intensity interval training (HIIT) format. The boot camp concept is savvy marketing that brings to mind high intensity, fitness gains, weight loss, and teamwork.

Goal-based programs such as boot camp and HIIT can attract a wide variety of participants, making it critical to have expert teaching skills (covered in more detail in chapters 6 and 7). Because these programs can include clients from beginner through expert, it is wise to offer multiple class levels to provide appropriate skill and intensity progressions and regressions. For instance, a 9:00 a.m. class on Monday, Wednesday, and Friday might be level 2 workouts, whereas Tuesday and Thursday at this time could be the introductory class time slot. This can allow for large differences in skill and fitness level, and letting clients graduate to higher levels gives them something to aim for.

On the other end of the spectrum, hospital-based fitness centers can provide a perfect setting for very specific group needs. Carol Lynne Teteak, MS, and fitness coordinator at Seven Bridges Edward-Elmhurst Health and Fitness Center in Woodridge, Illinois, works with many different groups. This facility offers three class size options of either three, four, or five to eight participants per group, with a higher price point for smaller groups. A minimum of six one-hour sessions are required. All hourly rates have two prices: one for members and one for nonmembers. Hospital-based facilities see all ages and populations and also work with groups with a need for specialized training, such as clients with Parkinson's disease and diabetes. They also may offer groups for fall prevention and sports injury prevention, as well as sports-specific programs like GolfSMART and RunSMART.

Who Participates in Small-Group Training?

From aggressive, high-intensity boot camp to gentle movement for the active older adult, an SGT instructor has a wide variety of choices of what type of exercise to offer, who to work with, and how to put them together in a marketable package. The most important decision to make initially is what population you'd like to work with. You may think that being specific will limit your business opportunities, but in fact it will not. First, you can more purposefully target your program design to the goals and needs of your clients if all have similar objectives. This is almost impossible to do when your group's goals are overly diversified. Although it's not always possible to separate newer folks from more advanced individuals, multilevel teaching and clear communication techniques can accommodate different fitness and skill levels within the same group class.

Targeting your group also allows you to purposefully direct your marketing. Different groups will respond to different marketing, so knowing exactly whom you'd like to train is an advantage. Whether it's women or men only, active older adults, adolescents, or athletes, having a clear focus will drive and center your efforts. For example, all-female classes, such as Strollercise for new moms, not only offer common training objectives, but also an element of socialization. Mothers of small children and infants are often socially isolated from adults and being around like-minded women can be a welcome experience.

Active older adults are also an ideal population to work with. If you do own a facility, offering classes at around 11:00 a.m.—typically a downtime for a studio—is perfect for this population. These groups also have similar goals and needs and are motivated by the appeal of socialization. Additionally, having a fixed income makes the price point of small-group training preferable to personal training and a smaller group makes it more personalized.

Weight-loss training may attract a more diverse group of people, but again, as long as the group objective is clear, you can develop a specific targeted program while also providing your clients with the social support of a group. It can help relieve the pain and shame many feel at the daunting prospect of starting a new exercise program when they feel they don't "look the part."

Equipment-focused groups such as kettlebell, suspension training, and Pilates Reformer classes are also extremely popular. These specific types of equipment demand specialized skills and attract unique groups that can build a successful business. Nico Gonzalez at Fitness Physiques by Nico G in Cincinnati, Ohio, has built a strong studio business based on equipment. Nico offers 16 Pilates equipment sessions per week for 3 to 5 clients per session, four Bodhi Suspension circuit training sessions per week for 4 to 10 clients per session, and two sessions per week of CoreAlign/Cycle for 3 to 4 clients per session. Nico specializes in workouts for special populations, including those with osteoporosis; hip, knee, or shoulder replacements and surgeries; and lower back disorders and neck and shoulder concerns.

In sum, targeting a client base will depend on your interests and your area of expertise. If you feel passionate about working with older populations or driven to get kids moving, then you will no doubt take the necessary steps towards educating yourself to best work with those groups. With so many possibilities, it's essential to work with the groups you feel most connected to.

In the Trenches

Phil Dozois, NASM CPT, PES, CES, IFS, and owner and founder of Breakthru Fitness in Pasadena, California, offers private and small-group training for members. Breakthru Fitness also offers a monthly SGT membership that allows members to book unlimited SGT sessions (booking is available online or through an app).

Phil adds that SGT appeals to two different types of clients: those who want direction and support, and those who want competition and challenge. There are several membership options allowing you to participate in groups of varying size. Depending on the size of the group, the price of the membership varies. Breakthru Fitness offers membership options for groups of 2 to 6 and 8 to 10, and provides designated areas for each.

Breakthru Fitness has a unique business model based on membership levels that provide unlimited access to SGT formats rather than session-based purchases. For example:

Level 1: Traditional group fitness classes + access to the club

Level 2: Large-group training (5-20 people) + traditional group fitness classes + access to the club

Level 3: Team training (unlimited SGT 8-10 people) + large-group training (5-20 people) + traditional group fitness classes + access to the club

Summary

Whether you build your group based on goals, populations, or style of training, the class needs to have goals that are clearly defined and specific to your clients. In chapters 6 and 7 you'll be learning how to work with groups, communicate effectively, and use multilevel teaching. In chapter 9 you will review all the training and programming principles necessary to build workouts specific to your groups' needs and goals. Throughout the book there are progressive programs to inspire and guide you. Not only will you learn to charismatically train your groups, you will also learn to build a business. When you have the knowledge, training is more than a job—it can be a passion! The career of your dreams can support you financially while also making a difference in the lives of the people you train.

CHAPTER 2

Risk Management and Safe Training Practices

Whether you own your own studio or you're an employee of a club or chain, it's important to consider your legal and professional responsibilities and have a risk-management plan in place. Maintaining safe training practices goes beyond having **CPR** and **AED** certifications; it is essential to have forethought and careful planning. This is especially true if you are a studio owner or have an outdoor boot camp business. If so, it is essential to familiarize yourself with your legal and professional responsibilities, understand liability and negligence, ensure your equipment is in perfect working order, and make sure your facility environment is suitable. For the SGT instructor who's working in a club setting, your areas of responsibility include health screening, fitness and exercise testing, programming, instruction, and supervision and appropriate use of equipment.

Liability and Negligence

Liability refers to your legal responsibility recognized in a court of law. Unfortunately, every time you stand in front of your groups, you are liable, meaning you are responsible for knowing the limitations of the individuals you're instructing. This responsibility is also known as a *standard of care* and must meet the current professional standards. When this quality of service is not met and an injury occurs as a result of negligence, a lawsuit may be the consequence. Negligence may be defined as "failure to use reasonable care, resulting in damage or injury to another" (Hobson, 2004, p. 292). Failure to use reasonable care or a failure to act refers to a task performed incorrectly or not performed. This means an SGT instructor could be sued not only for doing something incorrectly but also for failing to do something that would be expected within their scope of practice or responsibilities.

Areas of responsibility as an SGT instructor include far more than just exercise instruction. The following also fall into the category of responsibility:

- *Health screening*. Each participant should receive a thorough evaluation prior to starting an exercise program (see chapter 5).
- *Fitness and exercise testing*. This testing should be appropriate to the individual being tested, as well as valid, effective, and time efficient. The testing must be performed within your scope of practice according to your qualifications as a certified fitness instructor (see chapter 5).
- *Programming*. The consideration of health history is essential. Programs must follow accepted protocols appropriate to the individuals being trained (see chapter 9).

SCOPE OF PRACTICE

It's important to understand and be clear about what constitutes an instructor's scope of practice. Scope of practice can be defined as the following:

- *Legal range of services that professionals in a given field can provide.* As an SGT instructor, this means that you are qualified to teach classes.
- *Settings in which those services can be provided.* If you own a studio, then you are responsible for the safety within that space. If you're in a park or other outdoor area, then you are responsible for the area in which you teach. This makes your choice of training space an important one.
- *Laws, rules, and regulations that govern a profession and are established for the protection of the public.* These laws are in place to protect your participants from potential negligence.

The scope of practice indicates that, as a certified fitness professional, you are qualified to lead, instruct, or supervise exercise sessions for clients or classes. It also indicates that, unless otherwise qualified as a doctor, nurse, or physical therapist, you cannot diagnose or treat injuries. If a participant asks for medical or nutritional advice, it is prudent to suggest they contact their doctor or speak to a registered nutritionist. Only medical professionals can diagnose or treat injuries. Even something as simple as suggesting that an individual should ice an ankle injury could be misinterpreted if your instructions are not specific enough—for example, if the client goes home and puts ice on their ankle for an hour and gets frostbite, you may be liable. Although this may seem obvious to you as the instructor, it may not be to the person with the injury.

It's a complex issue, so taking a conservative approach is a good idea. This is especially true of suggesting dietary supplements. Only a doctor or medical professional can prescribe vitamins or even over-the-counter pain medication. Suggesting that your client speak to their doctor is the best practice.

Instruction and Demonstration

In terms of safety and risk management, instruction should adequately inform participants how an exercise should be safely performed. If a participant is injured as a result of poor instruction, you could be liable. In a court of law, your instruction would be assessed by an expert witness to judge whether your techniques are consistent with professionally recognized standards. Lack of adequate instruction can open the door to liability. Mastering essential teaching skills for effective instruction is covered in depth in chapter 7.

Supervision

As an SGT instructor, it is your responsibility to supervise all aspects of your class. Continuous supervision should be provided within the immediate proximity to the participant. The level of supervision must be consistent with your standard of care and should be adequate and proper. This includes consideration of your class size and environment. Having sufficient space for your participants to move is dependent on the type of class and movements being taught and may also vary with the population of the class—working with a group of strong athletes requires completely different levels of observation than with a group of deconditioned seniors. Supervision may also be specific to the activity a participant is performing. For example, kettlebells or medicine balls require excellent supervision. Swinging heavy metal objects while sweating, or throwing and catching a heavy ball, presents a whole set of challenges in terms of supervision and instruction. Watching your participants closely, keeping the floor clear of clutter, and helping your folks stay focused can all be helpful ways to optimize the supervision of your group.

Facilities

Opening your own studio space can be a wonderful but overwhelming experience. When it comes to legalities, safety is the priority. Even if you're only renting space in an existing studio, you are still responsible for making sure what you are doing is appropriate for the surface you're on, the amount of space you have for your group, and even lighting and visibility. The training surface is an immediate concern because impact and traction are major safety issues. Outdoor surfaces can present a different set of challenges. For example, if you're teaching a small group in a park in the early morning and the grass is wet and slick, rapid changes of direction could prove unsafe. Please refer to *ACSM's Health/Fitness Facility Standards and Guidelines, Fifth Edition,* for more information.

Equipment

If your program uses exercise equipment, your legal concerns involve their installation, maintenance, and repair, as well as selecting what's most appropriate for your particular groups. A thorough risk-management plan will consider that the equipment selected meets all safety and design standards within the industry, that the assembly of the equipment follows the manufacturers' guidelines, and that regular maintenance of that equipment is performed. SGT instructors should be aware that not all equipment is appropriate for all populations and that recommending specific equipment should be done cautiously. Be particularly alert to wear and tear of rubber resistance equipment and check regularly for any small tears or deterioration, which can be potentially dangerous if equipment becomes worn and snaps. It should be stored in a cool, dry area away from direct sunlight.

Accident Reporting

No matter how prepared you are, accidents that cause injury can happen during an exercise session. As an SGT instructor, it is your responsibility to file an accident report. This accident report should be retained for several years, depending on the statute of limitations in your area. If the accident occurred during the exercise session, a detailed written class plan should be included with the report. The following information should be included in your accident report:

- Name, address, and phone number of the injured person
- Time, date, and location where the accident occurred
- A concise description of the injury, the body part affected, and type of injury (i.e., "cut on the right palm of the hand")
- A description of the equipment used, including machine serial number, if applicable
- A description of the level of supervision and instruction being given at the time of the injury
- A brief and factual description of how the injury occurred with no opinions on fault or cause
- Names, addresses, and phone numbers of any witnesses
- A statement of any actions taken at the time of the injury, such as any first aid given, physician referral, or ambulance called
- Signatures of both the injured person and the supervisor

See figure 2.1 for a sample incident report form that you can copy for your personal use. When filling out this form, please make multiple copies for all involved, including the insurer, the individual involved in the incident, and the club's incident report files.

Figure 2.1   Incident report form

Date _____   Time of incident _____ a.m./p.m.

Name and contact information

Last name: _____   First name: _____   Middle initial: _____

Address: _____

City: _____   State: _____   Zip: _____

Phone number: _____   Email address: _____

Club details

Is injured party a club member? _____ YES _____ NO

Club name: _____

Club location: _____

Incident details

Hospital/EMS or physician notified? _____ YES _____ NO

Name of caller: _____   Time of initial call: _____

Time of any follow-up calls: _____

Time of EMS arrival: _____   Time of EMS departure: _____

Hospital taken to: _____   Name of EMS contact: _____

Description of the incident _____

_____

_____

_____

Skin broken? _____ YES _____ NO   Visible injury? _____ YES _____ NO

If eye injury, was eye protection being worn? _____ YES _____ NO

Was an AED used? _____ YES _____ NO   Was CPR applied? _____ YES _____ NO

Was first aid applied? _____ YES _____ NO   Did the police investigate? _____ YES _____ NO

If yes, please give name, rank, and contact information:

Name: _____

Position: _____   Contact: _____

Did another agency investigate (fire department)? _____ YES _____ NO

If yes, please give name, rank, and contact information:

Name: _____   Position: _____

Contact: _____

Report submitted by: _____

Signature: _____   Date and time submitted: _____

Witness: _____   Date and time submitted: _____

From K. Roberts, *A Professional's Guide to Small-Group Personal Training* (Champaign, IL: Human Kinetics, 2022).

RISK MANAGEMENT: KEEPING YOUR PARTICIPANTS SAFE

As a fitness leader or business owner, one of your most important duties includes successful risk management. More than just avoiding accidents or potential lawsuits, creating an environment that allows your groups to have an enjoyable experience while risks are kept to a minimum is a part of providing excellent customer service! Obvious hazards should be avoided, such as faulty, worn equipment or uneven turf during an outdoor class. You can further reduce risk by keeping in mind the type of participant and their needs and capabilities, along with a careful examination of the space, surface, and equipment.

You should also consider the risk-to-benefit ratio, which examines and quantifies the risk of an exercise versus the benefit derived from it. With almost any movement there can be a risk, even if it's a minute chance of injury. An exercise with a poor risk-to-benefit ratio has a high risk of injury with a low chance of benefit. No matter how good you think an exercise might be, the appropriateness and risks should always be a factor.

This is also where the importance of excellent teaching skills comes into play. A movement is only as good as how well it's performed, and an exercise is only effective if it's appropriate for the client performing it. For example, a deadlift is a great exercise when performed correctly but dangerous when performed incorrectly. Deadlifts are also not appropriate for everyone. When choosing an exercise, it should be effective, appropriate, and taught and performed correctly. The important thing to keep in mind is that for an exercise to be safe and effective, it needs to be taught at the correct level or modified to suit the level of the learner and coached in a way that enables them to be successful. This guarantees that you'll be on the right end of the risk-to-benefit ratio. Communication, coaching, and how people learn will be covered in more depth in chapter 7.

Emergency Response System

Having an emergency response system is critical for the safety of your participants and is fundamental to all gym and studio settings. Emergency policies, procedures, and practices for health and fitness facilities must never be neglected. All facilities offering exercise services are required to have written emergency response system policies and procedures that are reviewed and rehearsed regularly. Such policies enable training staff to handle basic first-aid situations as well as emergency events. There are several requirements for a studio's or gym's emergency response system:

- The system, including all emergency instructions and staff training, must be fully documented. These documents must be kept in an area that can be easily accessed by the staff.
- The system should identify an on-site coordinator. This individual is responsible for the overall level of emergency preparedness.
- Local health care or medical personnel should be consulted to help develop the emergency response program.

- All possible major emergency situations that may occur should be covered in the plan. This may include conditions such as hypoglycemia or common orthopedic injuries or severe events such as sudden cardiac arrest, myocardial infarction, or stroke. The system must also address other possible emergency situations such as fires, chemical accidents, or severe weather.

- The emergency response system must have a contingency plan that describes all steps and instructions for the various types of emergency and the roles each staff member will play.

- The location for all emergency exits and accessible telephones for calling 911 as well as contact information and all necessary steps for communicating with local emergency services must be clarified in the plan. The location and availability of first-aid kits and other medical equipment within the facility must also be included.

- The emergency response system must be reviewed and rehearsed twice yearly. This must be recorded in a logbook that includes when the rehearsals took place and who participated in them.

- All trainers or personnel involved in the exercise setting must be certified in basic cardiopulmonary resuscitation (CPR) and the use of automated external defibrillators (AED).

- All exercise facilities must have a publicly accessible AED. A skills and practice session with the AED should be reviewed every three to six months, along with regular monitoring and maintenance of the AED according to manufacturer's specification.

Once an emergency response system is written and implemented, the studio or gym becomes a safer environment for all clients and staff. This also provides the owner with a certain peace of mind, knowing risk has been minimized as much as possible.

Insurance

Depending on your business, you may need different levels and types of insurance. If, for example, you run your own studio, then you will need general liability insurance, professional liability insurance, and even an umbrella policy. For independent contractors, liability insurance against lawsuits is essential. Because your income relies on you being active as a full-time fitness professional, disability insurance can also be a good idea. Having the safety net of good insurance coverage can make all the difference if something does go wrong. Accidents can happen even with the best planning and being protected against financial losses can save your business. The following is an overview of the many different types of insurance you may need for your business:

- *General liability insurance.* This type of insurance is used by a facility to cover all basic "trip-and-fall" injuries.

- *Professional liability insurance.* This type of insurance covers all claims of negligence based on professional duties.

- *Disability insurance.* This type of insurance is important to protect you in case of injury and a loss of income.

- *Individual medical insurance.* This type of insurance is necessary for any type of medical coverage or hospitalization coverage.
- *An umbrella liability policy.* This is used to provide the insured with additional coverage in all insurance categories.

Waivers and Informed Consent

Utilizing a waiver or obtaining informed consent is extremely important and should be obligatory for every client. It's important to consider, however, that a waiver will not necessarily protect the instructor or fitness facility against a charge of negligence. Waivers must be clearly written to be effective and ideally include statements that participants waive all claims to damages, even those caused by negligence. Ideally, through careful assessments, good planning, and thoughtful teaching this will never need to be fought in a court of law.

It's essential that you obtain written consent prior to any assessment, exercise test, or participation in your classes. The form should notify the participant of any risks or benefits and also inform them that they are free to discontinue or withdraw from your groups at any time.

You may wish to consult with an attorney for local laws regarding fitness classes. For more in-depth guidance in this area, consult www.ihrsa.org/improve-your-club, where you'll find additional forms and information on specific standards, policies, and procedures for risk management. See figure 2.2 for a sample combined waiver and informed consent form.

Figure 2.2 Waiver and informed consent form

I agree to abide by the rules and regulations of the club/classes/services provided, including the completion of a pre-activity screening questionnaire and/or health/medical information questionnaire prior to participation in any physical activities at the club/studio/classes. Furthermore, I agree that all participation in classes, programs, and services shall be undertaken at my sole risk and the club shall not be liable for any injuries, accidents, or death occurring to me, including those resulting from the club's negligence arising either directly or indirectly out of my participation in classes or programs. I, for myself and on behalf of my executors, administrators, heirs, and assigns, do hereby expressly release, discharge, waive, relinquish, and covenant not to sue the studio or its affiliates, officers, directors, agents, instructors, trainers, or employees for all such claims, demands, injuries, damages, or causes of action, including those resulting from the club's/studio's/instructor's negligence, arising either directly or indirectly out of my participation in programs and services.

I declare that I have completed the club's pre-activity screening questionnaire and/or health/medical information questionnaire and that I am physically able to participate in physical activity. Furthermore, I acknowledge that the trainer has advised me to obtain a physician's clearance in the event the answers on either the pre-activity screening questionnaire and/or health/medical information questionnaire indicates that I should not participate in a program of physical activity without a physician's clearance beforehand.

Client signature: _____ Date: _____

Staff witness signature: _____

From K. Roberts, *A Professional's Guide to Small-Group Personal Training* (Champaign, IL: Human Kinetics, 2022).

Certifications

It is wise to stay current with your certification and education. By designing and running classes that are up to professional standards and implementing proper procedures for adequate supervision through all phases of the exercise program, risks can be attenuated. Keeping the facility free of hazards and maintaining sufficient space for each individual can further limit liability. As an employer, it is essential to require all instructors to have current CPR and AED training and certification. It is important to consider that professional standards continually evolve, and it is the responsibility of the instructor to stay up to date with legal requirements. By staying informed, SGT instructors can more successfully limit liability while maximizing client safety and enjoyment.

In the Trenches

Kristopher Kory, LMT, owner of and instructor for the past 10 years at Korlates Fitness in Avon, Connecticut, has always carried liability coverage as an instructor, presenter, and personal trainer, even before owning his own studio. According to Kris, "the thought of someone getting injured during my direction, even if it is of their own accord, is heartbreaking. Being taken to court can prove to be extremely costly. So protection is of the utmost importance, especially when you have a home and/or family to take care of."

The Korlates Fitness studio space is rented, and the landlord requires that Kris carry a certain dollar amount of liability insurance. In addition to that, Kris has extra insurance that would cover damage to his equipment and personal property by way of fire or theft, including broken window glass or water damage if the roof leaked or a pipe broke.

Kris also carries loss of income insurance in case he can't work if the studio is destroyed. Being fully covered includes damage insurance if one of his outside signs is damaged or destroyed. Additionally, he also has fire department service charge insurance. Even though Kris carries liability coverage for the studio, he also has a policy for protection when traveling and teaching at other locations.

Summary

This chapter is designed not to scare you but to inform and guide you about your legal responsibilities and the risk-management strategies that will help protect you and your business. No matter how well you plan, coach, and supervise, accidents can happen. Liability waivers and informed consent documents are designed to help protect you and your clients. Staying ahead of the game is an essential part of being a successful business owner, and taking the proper steps can make all the difference should an incident occur.

Creating Your Plan

With so many opportunities for SGT instructors, it's now time to narrow your choices. Do you want to work for a company as an employee, work for yourself as a business owner, or work as an independent contractor designing and teaching programs for other organizations? This chapter will cover the pros and cons of each.

Although employment status may vary, you will need to put together and implement a business plan. As the saying goes, if you fail to plan, you plan to fail! No one starts a business planning to fail, but trainers often fail to consider how they will run their day-to-day operations. You should have a well-organized business plan in place, including knowing your target client, understanding the market economy, and being aware of your competition.

Session Options for Your Business

Chapter 1 examined the different types of groups you can train; this chapter is going to help you put together a business plan. If you are going to run your own business, you have many decisions to make—for example, will you hold open sessions or closed sessions? Open sessions are simple to administer because they are drop in; people may come and go without committing to a specific number of classes. For closed sessions, clients pay up front to commit to a specific number of classes in a specific time frame. That time frame is up to you—it could be 4 to 8 weeks, or even up to 90 days for a summer boot camp. There are advantages and disadvantages to both of these plans. Let's take a look.

Open Sessions

The main advantage of open sessions is the ease of operation; people come and go at their convenience. All you need to do is decide on pricing, the types of packages available (price points for each number of classes), cancellation policy, and whether or not the classes need to be used within a specific time frame. Pricing and packages will be discussed later in this chapter, but one of the real advantages of open sessions is in having a more flexible cancellation policy. You will want to be extremely clear about your cancellation policy up front! There should be no surprises when it comes to cancellation fees. Make sure your clients know what to expect when it comes to no-shows and last-minute cancellations. If your program is heavily booked it's important to protect yourself from unreliability, so having a waitlist can be helpful.

Although people are coming at their convenience, you will still want them to book the class ahead of time so you can plan accordingly. Having an app or website for booking makes this simple. There are many apps and website templates available that can simplify how you administer your program. This makes your planning simple and also convenient for your clients.

The disadvantage is that open sessions don't allow for continuity and make it hard to have a progressive program. Without a prescribed number of sessions, assessments and reassessments are also difficult to handle. It also makes it a little harder to get to know people or build any real team cohesiveness. When you have the same people coming week-to-week, it's much easier to build camaraderie. Not only do you get to know your folks, they get to know each other and build friendships.

Closed Sessions

Closed sessions have some definite advantages, especially when you want to build a progressive program. When you train clients for a designated number of weeks, you have the opportunity to develop not only methodical movement progressions, but also stronger interpersonal relationships. Closed sessions also make it easier to build team rapport (further discussed in chapter 8). Assessments and exercise testing (see chapter 5) are also reasonably simple to administer in closed sessions. Even if individual assessments are not in your business model, a group exercise test can be performed during the first and last session, providing additional motivation. Seeing their results at the beginning and end is an effective way for a client to validate their investment.

There are some disadvantages to closed sessions, however. You will need to make some clear administrative decisions about inevitable no-shows and last-minute cancellations to determine what will work best for your business and also for your clients. A no-cancellation policy can motivate people to come when they don't feel like it, but you will need to make that rule extremely clear to avoid misunderstandings. Cancellations for illness and family emergencies are also factors to consider. No matter which type of sessions you run, how you handle last-minute cancellations needs to be up front and unambiguous. If you're working with online or app bookings, it's important to consider the loss of income for cancellations.

Regardless of whether you run open or closed sessions, you need to consider who will be your target audience, how long the sessions will run, and what will be the goal of the program. If it's a closed session, you will also need to decide how many weeks each program will run.

Addressing what makes your program unique helps market it. The name or theme of your program can spark interest; it can delineate you from your competitors and define what you're offering to your potential clients. Then, making it an incredible experience will build word of mouth and great retention.

The Business Plan

Establishing a successful SGT program requires the time to develop a comprehensive business plan with the purpose of defining the goals and creating an action plan. A business plan may include the following parts:

- Executive summary
- Market analysis
- Company description
- Organization and management
- Marketing and sales management
- Service
- Funding request
- Financials
- Appendix

Executive Summary

The executive summary is a brief outline of the company's purpose and goals and includes a brief description of products and services. It is the doorway to your business plan, an overview that summarizes the key points and strengths. This section appears first in the final business plan and highlights all other sections. For this reason, you may want to write it last. However, writing the executive summary first may help you bring focus to the rest of your plan. Either way can work well, but no matter what, this is critical to the overall scheme of your business.

Market Analysis

By identifying your target demographic and your competitors in the market, you'll distinguish your prospective customer base. It can also assist in maximizing the return on your marketing investment by helping you develop a plan to communicate directly with your target audience. When analyzing your market, it's important to consider the economic environment of your neighborhood. What are similar businesses charging for their services? What differentiates your company from the competition? Is it the workout itself, or are you providing a truly unique experience that goes beyond the physical classes? When you create a memorable experience, you no longer have to compete with anyone!

An analysis of strengths, weaknesses, opportunities, and threats (SWOT) can assist this process. A SWOT analysis is a traditional business practice that involves the evaluation of the relative strengths and weaknesses of your business in order to identify what you can build, improve, and grow. It can also help you develop your company description by defining your particular strengths and what differentiates you from your competition. By delineating your strengths you can better brand your services for marketing purposes; by identifying your weaknesses, you can address how to improve them and the overall administration of your business.

Strengths include how you construct and lead your actual workouts. You should incorporate your specific education, experience, specialization, and skills in your area of expertise. What types of services are you providing in addition to the classes? Consider amenities such as parking, showers, towels, lockers, and water and other beverages. Location, the cleanliness of your facility, your equipment, and staff can also be listed in your strengths.

You should also examine your weaknesses to see where you can make improvements. These may be related to your interpersonal skills, program design, or leadership (all covered in later chapters of this book). This also takes a straightforward appraisal of all the related services you are supplying. What skills can you improve on? What other services can you provide? What value can you add to your client's experience? It also entails looking at how you can be part of your community and how you can create community within your groups. How can you better engage your individuals to be more involved? Look for these opportunities to grow your existing services.

Threats can include other businesses in your local area, including big box gyms, especially if you're running a studio and the club is offering similar services as well as memberships. This is where you need to examine the level of service you are providing—people will be willing to come to you if you are offering an amazing experience. Threats may also include the economy in general. What are the financial restraints of your specific market? For example, active older adults may have a fixed income, so price will be a true concern of theirs. However, a threat can become an opportunity. Through close examination of your local competition, you will be able to see what they are missing and fill that void.

One more factor in your market analysis is considering the time of the day that holding classes would best suit your target demographic. Active older adults generally prefer to train in the midmorning; kids right after school; moms after dropping kids off at school; corporate fitness groups and other working adults before work, over lunch, and after work. You have many choices to make good use of your space, depending on the demographic you'd like to teach and space you'll be training in.

Company Description

Having a company description and a mission statement can help define your purpose. This also includes company goals and projected future services. For example, if you own a studio business and intend to expand and hire other trainers, this should be part of your plan. The company description will also help with any kind of funding request from banks or investors. The company description includes your qualifications and experience. Some questions you may want to ask yourself as you write a company description include: Who will run this business? Will you be the CEO? Will you have management or staff? If you plan on expanding, is there adjacent space available?

Organization and Management

If your goal is to start a company, then deciding which type of business structure is right for you is also an important factor. There are a lot of choices and opportunities. You may need to consult an attorney or accountant to get help setting up as a corporation. Never hesitate in getting the right kind of help—it is best to get started on the right footing.

Marketing and Sales Management

Marketing expenses can vary wildly, from costly commercials to free social media posts. However, word of mouth will always be your greatest marketing tool, and that only comes from providing an incredible experience. People talk! They may not remember what exercises you had them do, but they will always remember how you made them feel. It can be powerful to create a page on your website that includes clients' testimonials and before and after pictures, especially if your business involves weight loss. Your clients can be your greatest advocates.

Marketing through social media can be a double-edged sword. It can work incredibly well, but people are weary of being sold to, so it's best to avoid any hard selling. Tips for maximizing your social media for marketing are covered in detail in chapter 4. If social media is not on your agenda, then writing fitness or nutrition blogs can be another way to market and create a presence online. This can be especially useful to drive readers to your studio's website and potentially build business.

If you do decide to invest in some mainstream marketing, monitor it closely to see that you are in fact getting a good return. With a website, a blog, and social media, it's quite simple to see how well you're engaging people.

One important factor in marketing your business is to make sure you're consistent with your message. Your logo, website, brochures, and business cards should be consistent and cohesive. Branding and creating marketing that appeals to your target audience is critical, so be specific. One simple marketing tool is to create and sell branded apparel. T-shirts, caps, water bottles, and small workout towels are great ways to get your name in front of people. Again, the look of these should be consistent with your brand and who your potential clients will be.

If you're running a larger business, having a sales manager can take that stress off your plate. Trainers don't always make the best salespeople! You can also utilize your website or a variety of apps for class bookings and sales. This approach can dramatically simplify the process. With a great website you'll be able to market and sell sessions without needing face-to-face sales. Whether you decide to go with an app, a website, or direct salespeople may depend on the size of your business. Web design and hosting costs can be reasonable. Look online at what other businesses are doing and get a clear idea of how you'd like your site to look and whether you want to sell directly from your site. If it's a simple landing site without direct sales, it's something you can most likely do yourself.

Service

What specifications does your business require? What type of service will you be offering? Do you require a membership or is it pay-as-you-go? What type of setting will you be offering that service in? Here, you must decide what you're going to need. Whether you lease space for your own studio or rent space from another studio, private studio settings are always good environments for SGT classes. Typically, studios don't offer general memberships, so you're not competing for equipment with club members. If you are going to offer memberships, then it's best to have a designated space for your SGT sessions.

Important factors to consider before opening your own studio include how big your group is going to be, what kind of equipment you need, and what amenities will your service offer, such as towels and showers. Parks frequently require a permit to run a small group on public property, so check with your local parks and recreation department if you plan to work outdoors. If you own the business, adequate parking (whether street parking or a lot) is extremely important to include in your plan as well.

Funding Request

The funding request needs to include the costs for capital investment, which includes a lease, equipment, marketing, staffing, and everything in between. If you decide to find investors, then you will need to decide not only the amount of capital investment you need but also what investors will receive in return. What percentage of ownership and corresponding percentage of seats on the board of directors will you be willing to share?

Financials

When examining financials, another factor you'll want to consider is an industry overview. How much revenue do similar businesses produce in your region? Modeling your SGT business after similar successful companies is a way of creating an infrastructure for the direction you want to go.

Seasonal factors and holiday fluctuations can dramatically influence your business and should be accounted for. You may use it to your advantage with an outdoor summer bikini boot camp, for example, but if you don't have a backup plan for inclement weather you will need to know how to handle cancellations.

What will you charge and what are your costs? How much is your time worth to you? What is your projected weekly, monthly, and annual income? How much rent are you paying for your space? What are the expected fluctuations in your business due to holidays or seasons? These are all good questions to ask in your decision-making process. The key question is the first one, your costs versus what you will charge. Profits are the difference between the revenues collected and the expenses related to operating and delivering the program. Design a model to recognize all expenses and forecast your expected revenue in order to determine the long-term profitability of your business (see table 3.1 for an example of expenses and revenues for

TABLE 3.1   Expenses and Revenues for an Eight-Week SGT Program With Three Sessions per Week

Expenses		Revenue		
Item	Cost	Clients per session	Revenue $20 per session	Total profit or (loss)
Equipment*	$300.00	2	$40.00	**($56.25)**
Rent	$1,000.00	4	$80.00	**($16.25)**
Permits	0.00	6	$120.00	**$23.75**
Liability insurance	$50.00	8	$160.00	**$63.75**
Trainer compensation ($40 × 24 sessions)	$960.00			
Total	$2,310.00			
Expenses per session	$96.25			

*Once equipment is paid for, this is no longer an expense.

an eight-week program). This model can then assist you in forecasting how many sessions and people per session you will need in order to generate a profit.

One option is to offer an electronic funds transfer for ongoing memberships. This arrangement would be for an open session where the fees are collected electronically through a funds transfer directly to your business banking account. There are some specifics that must be defined in this type of arrangement. For example, it may include unlimited classes when classes are offered at various times of the day. This can be a successful model if you are targeting a specific population, such as corporate fitness, or utilizing a particular type of equipment, like suspension training or kettlebells.

If you are going to employ instructors to teach for you, you will need to decide on the type of compensation model. A flat fee would pay your instructor a particular amount of money regardless of the number of people in the class. If the goal is to keep your classes small and exclusive, this would be a fair practice. For the scaled fee, the instructor would receive a base plus a per-head amount. This incentivizes the instructor to build their classes.

Appendix

The appendix includes information about you and your instructors, including your experience, certifications, formal education and degrees, and any relevant continuing education.

In the Trenches

Robin Dayer, owner of Burn Studio in Conway, Arkansas, believes that creating a solid business model is one of the most important factors in the work done before the opening. "Knowing who you are and what you want to offer is key. For example, I knew that I wanted Burn to be known for having that small studio feel yet offer everything, much like in a big gym." This unique business offers four studio rooms under one roof, making a wide variety of offerings possible and creating a studio feel.

Memberships are sold for periods of 3, 6, or 12 months, which encourages regular commitment and helps with accountability. Payments for these membership options are done by automatic draft. Dayer values these automatic-draft memberships because they give "knowledge of what sort of revenue to expect for a given month." Members also have the option of getting monthly memberships, signing up for class packs, or purchasing just a single class. "We wanted to give them every option possible to attend class with us. In Conway, where we are located, we are on the higher-priced end of fitness offerings." To boost retention and referrals, Robin gives each new client a welcome bag with a water bottle and free class passes to share with a friend, plus a discount card for the first purchase of a month's membership.

During the COVID-19 pandemic, Burn Studio rebuilt their entire model and simplified pricing options due to new virtual needs. The business now offers three tiers: premium (or all access), livestreaming only, and on-demand only. According to Dayer, "We have found our best marketing always comes from social media. Ads on Instagram and Facebook have always proven successful. Instagram stories bring customers in; some end up becoming regular members."

Summary

Many instructors and trainers are great at coaching and supervising but not so good at running a business. This chapter has provided some easy-to-follow steps to set up your business and implement some systems to keep it running. As the saying goes: If you fail to plan, you plan to fail! Setting up a solid business foundation is like allowing a tree to grow deeper roots—you'll be more likely to weather any storms when your foundation is stronger.

CHAPTER 4

Building Your Client Base

Getting new clients is one of the most expensive things you can do to grow your business. Without a doubt, referrals and word of mouth are your two greatest tools for building your client base. It's far easier to retain a client than find a new one, and once you have a satisfied client, they are a source of possible referrals and good word of mouth. Therefore, building your client base means you also need to focus on retaining your existing client base. Poor retention will drive your business into the ground. Once you get a client, you simply can't afford to lose them! Some studies reveal that by increasing customer retention by as little as 5 percent, companies can potentially increase profits from 25 to 100 percent.

Investing in retention, developing a system for referrals, and utilizing cost-effective marketing are just some of the ways to build your client base. Unpredictability of income can plague an SGT business if these measures are not in place. This chapter will explore and expand on strategies to build a client base and ultimately create a business with a steady income.

Retention

If you're truly serious about building your business through high levels of retention, then world-class customer service should be your goal. Providing an unforgettably positive experience creates happy clients. Happy clients refer friends and family—in fact, a happy client will refer anyone who'll listen!

Training is a relational business. It involves having good rapport, developing trust and empathy, and understanding your client's needs and concerns. That initial rapport can be established through shared interests. What do you and your prospective client have in common? Finding shared interests can help develop trust. Remember, a one-sided relationship will not survive—you have to genuinely care about and want to help everyone in your group. From start to finish you have to work to help them achieve their goals. Your clients need to know that your concern goes beyond what they are paying you.

You can demonstrate your care for your clients through some simple actions. These also add value, which is an advantage in a competitive market. Here are some suggestions for enhancing your SGT class retention:

- Monthly printed newsletters
- Weekly emailed newsletters
- Blogs
- Recognition, such as plaques and awards for special efforts
- Educational audio or video for specific goals
- Water bottles, towels, T-shirts, and caps with your logo
- Birthday and Christmas cards
- Thank-you cards
- Gift cards or discounts for referrals

Referrals

The greatest compliment a client can give you is a referral. People trust the recommendation of a friend, family member, or colleague over someone unfamiliar with a sharp marketing plan. Learning to ask your clients to refer potential participants to your classes is not necessarily easy to do, but it can have an immediate and lasting effect on your business. Because there's no marketing expense for a referral, a new client is coming with only a positive, trusted endorsement.

However, it's not enough to be great at what you do and assume the result will be automatic referrals. Getting referrals requires a conscious effort and an effective system. Random acts, at best, get random results. In today's inconsistent, distracted, competitive marketplace, you cannot afford to sit back and wait for a client to refer someone to your classes. The following concrete system will entice your existing clients to help build your business:

- Give, then receive
- Enlist the power of numbers
- Create connection and relationships
- Build trust

Give, Then Receive

Reciprocity is a social norm of responding to an action with a similar action (either positive or negative). In terms of marketing, this works by giving a potential customer something of value in an attempt to prompt them to respond in kind. A good example is a free sample at the supermarket, which is not only an opportunity to try something, but an invitation to engage in the rule of reciprocity. Many people find it difficult to simply accept the free sample and walk away, and will instead buy the product (Fehr & Gächter, 2000). In the case of asking for a referral, a client is more likely to recommend you because they enjoy your sessions. For you as a trainer, part of your "giving" to your clients is the experience you create in your classes.

The other part can be in the form of an offer in order to incentivize referrals. You might give a discount on the next package of sessions or offer a gift card or branded merchandise. Logically, people always like to get a discount, so not only are they motivated to refer others, this could also provide incentive for them to sign up again. Offering discounts to first-time buyers is another good way to lower barriers. Sliding scales on prices for different package sizes or monthly memberships can provide the stability your business needs.

Make getting that referral more enticing. Offer a special deal to the referring client *and* the person being referred. This is where merchandise can come in handy. Offering T-shirts, caps, water bottles, or towels for the referral can be persuasive to the existing client, and a free trial class motivates the prospective participant.

Enlist the Power of Numbers

If every client could refer just one person, you could exponentially increase your customer base. Referral marketing is a path for building trust with new customers. Because there is an existing connection between you and your new customers, it makes people more likely to consider signing up with you. Word of mouth is the primary factor behind a good percentage of purchasing decisions, so it is wise to find ways to make this easier! Consider events such as "Bring Your Partner for Free" on Valentine's Day, or family and friends open house gatherings with free mini-classes and snacks. Providing opportunities for social events or special themed workouts are all ways to get people in the door and broaden your visibility within your community.

CREATING COMMUNITY

When building your classes, grouping people by specific goals and training objectives can also create community. Not only is it easier to write an effective program, it fosters relationships and socialization among the participants. Interactive games can further socialization: A fun one is to have people work with a partner for a drill or exercise set. Have them introduce themselves and then tell their partner their childhood nickname, then switch partners for each new exercise. For each exercise set, add some other rapport builder, such as the following:

- What's your favorite animal?
- What's your favorite food?
- What's your least favorite food?
- What's your favorite sport or team?
- What's number one on your bucket list?
- Where were you born?
- How many brothers and sisters do you have?

Having clients get to know each other can help increase group retention by fostering stronger relationships between team members. This element in training groups should not be overlooked. Building bonds between your folks can help with accountability. Getting and keeping people involved in the group through partner exercises and games adds a sense of fun while at the same time building connections.

Create Connection and Relationships

If you want to maximize your referrals, perhaps the most critical piece of the puzzle is having your clients connect with you. Creating connections with and among clients builds loyalty. Finding common ground can be a way of doing this. For example, if you enjoy tennis and your prospective client's goal is to improve their tennis game, an easy discussion about the sport can build rapport. So how do you have the clients in your class build loyalty to not just you, but also to the other people in the group? Create opportunities for your group to feel like they are working toward a common objective and that they can only get there through teamwork. Teamwork begins with your people getting to know each other. When you play team-building games, include your own answers so they get to know you as well as each other. This humanizes you and builds further connection between you and your clients.

Dan S. Kennedy (2013), a published business coach and consultant, shares that "if you want the highest possible retention and referrals, you will work at having your customers feel that they are in a relationship with you, not just a paying customer." In practice, this initial rapport is built in the first meeting, whether that's through email, over the phone, or in person. Your initial meeting should involve a "getting to know your potential client" phase. This also means having them get to know you!

Build Trust

The building of trust is critical in your client–instructor relationship. People crave trust, and once the foundation is built, it's hard for a competitor to break. This foundation begins with empathy, warmth, and genuineness, and when it's solid, it generates referrals. The relationship between instructor and participant is one of trust at the highest level. Clients come to you with some of their most personal insecurities. They often share intimate secrets about how they feel about themselves and their bodies, which they may have never even told their doctors. Being a trustworthy coach and an inspiring instructor requires high levels of integrity.

The number one objective for the development of trust is to remove or reduce the participant's sense of risk or uncertainty, thereby providing confidence and security. This is done through expert instruction and excellent communication—not only in your ability to speak, but also listen. If the client feels you understand their goals or have experience in helping people reach similar goals, you will build their trust.

Reinforce, Reach, and Return

To reinforce your marketing efforts, it's time to enhance your reach and increase your return. Lead boxes, charitable donations, word of mouth, partnerships, and community marketing can all broaden your influence within your community, thereby growing deeper roots to build a more solid foundation for your business.

Lead Box

A lead box is a fairly straightforward way to receive contact information from potential clients. You might, for example, provide free classes to the owner of a nearby organic café, and in return they place a jar next to the cash register

USING SOCIAL MEDIA TO BUILD YOUR BUSINESS

Because basic social media is free to use, maximizing the time you spend building an online presence is important. Social media can be extremely effective, but it can also be a huge time drain when used incorrectly. Amanda Vogel, a social media consultant for the fitness industry and blogger who reviews health and fitness products and technology, shares the following wisdom and experience.

What are your top three tips for marketing an SGT business on social media?

1. *Begin with a plan.*

It's tempting to post to social media only when you think of it. It's OK to post spontaneously sometimes, but using social media for marketing and business works best when you create a strategy that includes a long-range vision for what you will post and when you will post it—and why.

2. *Look past follower numbers.*

Gone are the days when all that mattered on social media was how many followers you had. In fact, focusing too much on follower numbers is considered outdated— one reason is because it's very easy to just buy fake followers. What matters more from a business perspective is how people engage with your content online and, ultimately, how well your social marketing makes a positive impact on your offline business. For best results, create content with your followers in mind. Focus on what's important to them—not what *you* think should be important to them.

3. *Be prepared to adapt.*

Social media changes often and quickly. What worked six months ago might not work as well now—that's just the nature of social media algorithms and people's fickle preferences online. While it's important to stay on top of new social features and trends, don't feel like you have to do it all. Choose your top two or three performing platforms and focus most of your efforts on those. Experiment with the content types (photos, videos, etc.) that generate the best responses.

What are your top three things to avoid?

1. *Avoid winging it.*

It's fine to put up a mishmash of posts on a personal page if you're using it just for fun. But when you're using social media to market your small-group training services, every post should have a specific goal that leads, in some way, back to your main goals for the business.

2. *Avoid veering off brand.*

Like it or not, sometimes the posts that get the highest engagement are silly at best and questionable or offensive at worst. Don't sacrifice your business's image just for the sake of getting more likes, comments, and shares. Always consider your business goals when posting to help you stay true to your brand.

3. *Avoid discouraging or careless posts.*

Anything you put on social media can make a lasting impression (good or bad), even if you delete it later. Keep your followers' best interests in mind. Post positive and thoughtful comments and images designed to motivate—not discourage—clients and prospective clients.

advertising your studio. Café customers put their business cards in the jar for a chance to win a free class with you. You, in return, receive leads, supplying you with opportunities to market your business. A lead box might be used at a café or restaurant, but it also could be at your hairdresser's salon or even your massage therapist clinic. Consider your target audience!

Rather than immediately sending hard-sell marketing to your leads, send a link to your educational blog or newsletter. With a soft-sell approach you again create reciprocity by first giving something to the prospective client without asking for something in return.

Charitable Donations

A great way to increase your community presence is to donate a class session to a local charity auction. Put together a nice package, including any printed marketing material, a professional-looking gift certificate, and a picture frame for the auction table with before and after pictures of your participants. You'll get a new face in your classes and increase your neighborhood presence while also raising money for charity.

Word of Mouth

Generating positive word-of-mouth referrals is and always will be the result of providing your groups with a consistently excellent experience. Exceptional experience starts with the four Ps: preparation, punctuality, professionalism, and personality. Get these to align and you have a good chance of making your business successful.

Partnerships

Strategic partnerships offer another opportunity to build your SGT business. For example, partnering with a company that delivers calorie-controlled meals for weight loss is a chance to not only help your clients improve body composition, but also double your clientele. As a partnership, you could share client contact information for marketing. This strategy is made far more effective if you include before and after pictures and testimonials from your groups. This can be done either with printed materials or on your website.

Another great opportunity for partnerships is through physical therapy clinics or chiropractic practices. Working and developing good relationships with the medical community is an excellent way to build credibility with potential clients. However, you first need to establish a reputation of excellence in your specialty and a sound relationship with the doctor, physical therapist, or chiropractor you're working with. Having the appropriate credentials and knowing your market are both critical factors.

Community Marketing

Athletic fundraising events may provide an excellent opportunity to market your business or yourself. You could even choose a charity, create your own event, and have your participants help with the fundraising, which in turn markets your classes. You can also find an event such as a fundraising walk, run, golf tournament, or bike ride. Many of these events provide training workouts to help build participants' fitness and prep them specifically for the challenge.

Try reaching out to the organizers and offer stretch, core, or injury prevention clinics for free. This type of outreach can set you up for success because your participants already have common objectives, thereby simplifying marketing, program design, and group coherence.

Any exposure to the already active market is like picking low-hanging fruit. Those who are already involved in activity might be looking for some performance advantages that you can provide through core training or injury prevention. Local fun runs or walks often do warm-ups for participants, which can be the perfect opportunity to connect with new faces. Charity and athletic events often have trade shows where you could offer one-on-one stretching or demonstrations in myofascial release techniques. Although it may cost a few dollars to participate, it's a good opportunity to get your name in front of people who are already active. This is especially valuable if you're doing sports-specific training for that activity.

In the Trenches

Nabil Mardini, co-owner of DIG Cycle and Strength in Los Angeles, California, offers indoor cycling and SGT TRX classes. He shares that "our market is for all those who are fit, looking to get back in shape, who are athletes, or who simply like to stay in shape. DIG caters to all women and men over the age of 18." Mardini is building his business through direct marketing, Groupon, Conejo Deals, social media (Facebook and Instagram), and TAF (Tell A Friend). Mardini encourages the DIG instructors to promote the studio and classes on their personal pages as well. DIG Cycle and Strength offers a free cycling and TRX class for first-time members. They also offer a $21 unlimited deal that is valid for one week from the day of purchase.

Summary

Ultimately, successful SGT instructors provide their clients with an incredible experience. Happy, loyal clients lead to referrals, which lead to a flourishing business. It cannot be overstated: Your ability to connect and build relationships with your clients is the foundation to the development of trust. Giving before expecting anything in return creates reciprocity, which in turn allows you to "soft sell" your classes. Creating a presence in your community through charitable service establishes your reputation and further builds trust. Working to build strategic relationships grows deeper roots for your business, benefiting you, your community, and your clients. Running a business is hard work, but if you're passionate about what you do, you'll find it's not just a way to make money, it can bring you purpose!

PART II

WORKING WITH SMALL GROUPS

CHAPTER 5

Assessment and Exercise Testing

Assessments allow you, as the trainer, to capture a snapshot of your client's current physical, mental, and emotional condition. Through assessments, you can set a baseline that allows you to gauge progression, which adds a great deal of value to your services and sets you apart from traditional group fitness classes, where formal assessments are rarely performed. These tests also direct your program design: Having a goal is a major component to program design, and exercise testing provides the start point.

How you structure your program is also going to influence the types of assessments you perform. For a four-week closed session, then a reasonably detailed assessment is a good idea (the PAR-Q+ along with some—or all—of the tests outlined in this chapter are a great place to start). Including some exercise testing along with assessments can help motivate your clients and ultimately build your business. If you're working with drop-in open sessions, then a PAR-Q+ or some form of health risk assessment is a minimum.

Health Risk Assessment

The health benefits of regular physical activity have been well documented and include improved cholesterol, lower blood pressure, reduced body fat, and increased cardiovascular fitness, just to name a few. Nonetheless, a health risk assessment (HRA) must be performed on anyone who will be training with you, regardless of their age or gender. The omission of this type of assessment can lead to serious health and legal implications.

An HRA is essential for the safety of your clients and is a vital first step in the relationship you will build. Because the HRA identifies the signs and symptoms suggestive of cardiovascular, pulmonary, and metabolic disease, it will distinguish any individual who should undergo a medical evaluation and exercise testing prior to initiating an exercise program. It can also identify individuals who should be excluded from exercise or physical activity until those conditions are corrected or under control, or who should exercise in a medically controlled environment.

Generally speaking, exercise does not provoke cardiovascular events in healthy individuals with normal cardiovascular systems. The risk of sudden cardiac death (SCD) or acute myocardial infarction (AMI) is very low in individuals performing low- to moderate-intensity exercise; however, there is an increased risk in individuals performing vigorous-intensity exercise, particularly in sedentary men and women. It has been documented that the increase in intensity and corresponding elevation in heart rate and systolic blood pressure may cause cracking in atherosclerotic plaques (fatty deposits inside the artery wall that are made up of cholesterol, cellular waste products, calcium, and fibrin) with resulting acute thrombosis, or blood clot within a blood vessel that obstructs blood flow. When a blood vessel is injured, the body uses platelets (thrombocytes) and fibrin to form a blood clot to prevent blood loss. The blood clots present a huge risk for AMI or stroke and can therefore be potentially deadly (ACSM, 2017).

A commonly used HRA form, called the Physical Activity Readiness Questionnaire for Everyone (PAR-Q+), is a safe preexercise screening measure for low- to moderate-intensity exercise (although not vigorous training). It serves as a minimal HRA prerequisite and is quick, easy, and noninvasive to administer. The PAR-Q+ is a good example of the type of critical initial screening to employ before you start to work with your clients. See figure 5.1 on pages 40-43 for the PAR-Q+.

Apparently healthy participants who do not currently exercise and have no history or symptoms of cardiovascular, metabolic, or renal disease can immediately, and without medical clearance, initiate an exercise program of light to moderate intensity. Participants who are already exercising regularly and have no history, signs, or symptoms can continue at their current levels of intensity and progress as appropriate (ACSM, 2017). Should your clients have a medical history or signs or symptoms suggestive of cardiovascular or metabolic disease, medical clearance should be gained prior to training. Even if your clients are already engaged in some form of regular training, an HRA must be performed for liability purposes. Should someone in your group experience a cardiovascular complication and you haven't conducted a PAR-Q+ or other HRA, you may be liable.

Fitness Assessment

It can be useful to perform a fitness assessment for your clients before they join your SGT program. It collects baseline data in order to develop a more personalized program and allows you to measure progress. This can be one of the delineating factors between SGT and group fitness classes, as group fitness classes rarely use assessments. Assessment also helps identify areas of health or injury risk the client may not be aware of, which can be compared to normative data for age and gender. This in turn can help motivate them into further action.

Some of the physiological assessments you should be familiar with and qualified to administer include the following:

- Resting heart rate
- Resting blood pressure
- Joint flexibility and muscle length

- Muscular endurance and strength
- Cardiorespiratory fitness
- Body composition
- Balance and core function
- Skill-related parameters (i.e., agility, coordination, power, reactivity, and speed)

Not all clients will need the same fitness assessments. Assessments should be specific to the needs and goals of the client. For example, if weight loss is a goal, then being competent at performing body composition assessments is critical. Whether you use skinfold calipers, a bioimpedance analysis device, or a tape measure for anthropometric data, being accurate and consistent is the key. If you're working with older populations, then muscular endurance, balance and core function, and resting vital signs are valuable. For athletes, having the appropriate test for their sport can make an impact on how you're going to train them. Regardless of who you train, always remember the one mandatory component is the health risk assessment to determine your client's cardiovascular risk and readiness for the correct intensity of activity.

It is important to be explicit in your instructions for assessments. Having clearly written instructions and a description of what to expect can help increase the test validity. When retesting is performed, the exact same instructions should be followed. Here are some basic suggestions for preliminary instructions, which may vary based on the type of test to be performed.

- Participants should refrain from ingesting food, alcohol, or caffeine or using tobacco products within three hours of testing.
- Participants should be rested for the assessment, avoiding significant exertion or exercise on the day of the testing.
- Clothing should permit freedom of movement and include appropriate footwear.
- Participants should drink ample fluids over the 24-hour period preceding the exercise test to ensure normal hydration.

2020 PAR-Q+

The Physical Activity Readiness Questionnaire for Everyone

The health benefits of regular physical activity are clear; more people should engage in physical activity every day of the week. Participating in physical activity is very safe for MOST people. This questionnaire will tell you whether it is necessary for you to seek further advice from your doctor OR a qualified exercise professional before becoming more physically active.

GENERAL HEALTH QUESTIONS

Please read the 7 questions below carefully and answer each one honestly: check YES or NO.	YES	NO
1) Has your doctor ever said that you have a heart condition ☐ OR high blood pressure ☐ ?	☐	☐
2) Do you feel pain in your chest at rest, during your daily activities of living, OR when you do physical activity?	☐	☐
3) Do you lose balance because of dizziness OR have you lost consciousness in the last 12 months? Please answer NO if your dizziness was associated with over-breathing (including during vigorous exercise).	☐	☐
4) Have you ever been diagnosed with another chronic medical condition (other than heart disease or high blood pressure)? PLEASE LIST CONDITION(S) HERE: _____	☐	☐
5) Are you currently taking prescribed medications for a chronic medical condition? PLEASE LIST CONDITION(S) AND MEDICATIONS HERE: _____	☐	☐
6) Do you currently have (or have had within the past 12 months) a bone, joint, or soft tissue (muscle, ligament, or tendon) problem that could be made worse by becoming more physically active? Please answer NO if you had a problem in the past, but it **does not limit your current ability** to be physically active. PLEASE LIST CONDITION(S) HERE: _____	☐	☐
7) Has your doctor ever said that you should only do medically supervised physical activity?	☐	☐

☑ **If you answered NO to all of the questions above, you are cleared for physical activity.**
Please sign the PARTICIPANT DECLARATION. You do not need to complete Pages 2 and 3.

▶ Start becoming much more physically active – start slowly and build up gradually.

▶ Follow Global Physical Activity Guidelines for your age (https://apps.who.int/iris/handle/10665/44399).

▶ You may take part in a health and fitness appraisal.

▶ If you are over the age of 45 yr and NOT accustomed to regular vigorous to maximal effort exercise, consult a qualified exercise professional before engaging in this intensity of exercise.

▶ If you have any further questions, contact a qualified exercise professional.

PARTICIPANT DECLARATION
If you are less than the legal age required for consent or require the assent of a care provider, your parent, guardian or care provider must also sign this form.

I, the undersigned, have read, understood to my full satisfaction and completed this questionnaire. I acknowledge that this physical activity clearance is valid for a maximum of 12 months from the date it is completed and becomes invalid if my condition changes. I also acknowledge that the community/fitness center may retain a copy of this form for its records. In these instances, it will maintain the confidentiality of the same, complying with applicable law.

NAME _____ DATE _____

SIGNATURE _____ WITNESS _____

SIGNATURE OF PARENT/GUARDIAN/CARE PROVIDER _____

⬤ **If you answered YES to one or more of the questions above, COMPLETE PAGES 2 AND 3.**

⚠ **Delay becoming more active if:**

✓ You have a temporary illness such as a cold or fever; it is best to wait until you feel better.

✓ You are pregnant - talk to your health care practitioner, your physician, a qualified exercise professional, and/or complete the ePARmed-X+ at www.eparmedx.com before becoming more physically active.

✓ Your health changes - answer the questions on Pages 2 and 3 of this document and/or talk to your doctor or a qualified exercise professional before continuing with any physical activity program.

Copyright © 2020 PAR-Q+ Collaboration 1 / 4
01-11-2019

FIGURE 5.1 Physical Activity Readiness Questionnaire for Everyone (PAR-Q+).

Reprinted with permission from the PAR-Q+ Collaboration and the authors of the PAR-Q+ (Dr. Darren Warburton, Dr. Norman Gledhill, Dr. Veronica Jamnik, and Dr. Shannon Bredin).

2020 PAR-Q+

FOLLOW-UP QUESTIONS ABOUT YOUR MEDICAL CONDITION(S)

1. **Do you have Arthritis, Osteoporosis, or Back Problems?**

If the above condition(s) is/are present, answer questions 1a-1c   If **NO** ☐ go to question 2

1a.	Do you have difficulty controlling your condition with medications or other physician-prescribed therapies? (Answer **NO** if you are not currently taking medications or other treatments)	YES ☐ NO ☐
1b.	Do you have joint problems causing pain, a recent fracture or fracture caused by osteoporosis or cancer, displaced vertebra (e.g., spondylolisthesis), and/or spondylolysis/pars defect (a crack in the bony ring on the back of the spinal column)?	YES ☐ NO ☐
1c.	Have you had steroid injections or taken steroid tablets regularly for more than 3 months?	YES ☐ NO ☐

2. **Do you currently have Cancer of any kind?**

If the above condition(s) is/are present, answer questions 2a-2b   If **NO** ☐ go to question 3

2a.	Does your cancer diagnosis include any of the following types: lung/bronchogenic, multiple myeloma (cancer of plasma cells), head, and/or neck?	YES ☐ NO ☐
2b.	Are you currently receiving cancer therapy (such as chemotherapy or radiotherapy)?	YES ☐ NO ☐

3. **Do you have a Heart or Cardiovascular Condition? This includes Coronary Artery Disease, Heart Failure, Diagnosed Abnormality of Heart Rhythm**

If the above condition(s) is/are present, answer questions 3a-3d   If **NO** ☐ go to question 4

3a.	Do you have difficulty controlling your condition with medications or other physician-prescribed therapies? (Answer **NO** if you are not currently taking medications or other treatments)	YES ☐ NO ☐
3b.	Do you have an irregular heart beat that requires medical management? (e.g., atrial fibrillation, premature ventricular contraction)	YES ☐ NO ☐
3c.	Do you have chronic heart failure?	YES ☐ NO ☐
3d.	Do you have diagnosed coronary artery (cardiovascular) disease and have not participated in regular physical activity in the last 2 months?	YES ☐ NO ☐

4. **Do you currently have High Blood Pressure?**

If the above condition(s) is/are present, answer questions 4a-4b   If **NO** ☐ go to question 5

4a.	Do you have difficulty controlling your condition with medications or other physician-prescribed therapies? (Answer **NO** if you are not currently taking medications or other treatments)	YES ☐ NO ☐
4b.	Do you have a resting blood pressure equal to or greater than 160/90 mmHg with or without medication? (Answer **YES** if you do not know your resting blood pressure)	YES ☐ NO ☐

5. **Do you have any Metabolic Conditions? This includes Type 1 Diabetes, Type 2 Diabetes, Pre-Diabetes**

If the above condition(s) is/are present, answer questions 5a-5e   If **NO** ☐ go to question 6

5a.	Do you often have difficulty controlling your blood sugar levels with foods, medications, or other physician-prescribed therapies?	YES ☐ NO ☐
5b.	Do you often suffer from signs and symptoms of low blood sugar (hypoglycemia) following exercise and/or during activities of daily living? Signs of hypoglycemia may include shakiness, nervousness, unusual irritability, abnormal sweating, dizziness or light-headedness, mental confusion, difficulty speaking, weakness, or sleepiness.	YES ☐ NO ☐
5c.	Do you have any signs or symptoms of diabetes complications such as heart or vascular disease and/or complications affecting your eyes, kidneys, **OR** the sensation in your toes and feet?	YES ☐ NO ☐
5d.	Do you have other metabolic conditions (such as current pregnancy-related diabetes, chronic kidney disease, or liver problems)?	YES ☐ NO ☐
5e.	Are you planning to engage in what for you is unusually high (or vigorous) intensity exercise in the near future?	YES ☐ NO ☐

Copyright © 2020 PAR-Q+ Collaboration   2 / 4
11-01-2019

(continued)

FIGURE 5.1 *(continued)*

Reprinted with permission from the PAR-Q+ Collaboration and the authors of the PAR-Q+ (Dr. Darren Warburton, Dr. Norman Gledhill, Dr. Veronica Jamnik, and Dr. Shannon Bredin).

2020 PAR-Q+

6.   Do you have any Mental Health Problems or Learning Difficulties? This includes Alzheimer's, Dementia, Depression, Anxiety Disorder, Eating Disorder, Psychotic Disorder, Intellectual Disability, Down Syndrome

If the above condition(s) is/are present, answer questions 6a-6b   If **NO** ☐ go to question 7

6a.	Do you have difficulty controlling your condition with medications or other physician-prescribed therapies? (Answer **NO** if you are not currently taking medications or other treatments)	YES ☐ NO ☐
6b.	Do you have Down Syndrome **AND** back problems affecting nerves or muscles?	YES ☐ NO ☐

7.   Do you have a Respiratory Disease? This includes Chronic Obstructive Pulmonary Disease, Asthma, Pulmonary High Blood Pressure

If the above condition(s) is/are present, answer questions 7a-7d   If **NO** ☐ go to question 8

7a.	Do you have difficulty controlling your condition with medications or other physician-prescribed therapies? (Answer **NO** if you are not currently taking medications or other treatments)	YES ☐ NO ☐
7b.	Has your doctor ever said your blood oxygen level is low at rest or during exercise and/or that you require supplemental oxygen therapy?	YES ☐ NO ☐
7c.	If asthmatic, do you currently have symptoms of chest tightness, wheezing, laboured breathing, consistent cough (more than 2 days/week), or have you used your rescue medication more than twice in the last week?	YES ☐ NO ☐
7d.	Has your doctor ever said you have high blood pressure in the blood vessels of your lungs?	YES ☐ NO ☐

8.   Do you have a Spinal Cord Injury? This includes Tetraplegia and Paraplegia

If the above condition(s) is/are present, answer questions 8a-8c   If **NO** ☐ go to question 9

8a.	Do you have difficulty controlling your condition with medications or other physician-prescribed therapies? (Answer **NO** if you are not currently taking medications or other treatments)	YES ☐ NO ☐
8b.	Do you commonly exhibit low resting blood pressure significant enough to cause dizziness, light-headedness, and/or fainting?	YES ☐ NO ☐
8c.	Has your physician indicated that you exhibit sudden bouts of high blood pressure (known as Autonomic Dysreflexia)?	YES ☐ NO ☐

9.   Have you had a Stroke? This includes Transient Ischemic Attack (TIA) or Cerebrovascular Event

If the above condition(s) is/are present, answer questions 9a-9c   If **NO** ☐ go to question 10

9a.	Do you have difficulty controlling your condition with medications or other physician-prescribed therapies? (Answer **NO** if you are not currently taking medications or other treatments)	YES ☐ NO ☐
9b.	Do you have any impairment in walking or mobility?	YES ☐ NO ☐
9c.	Have you experienced a stroke or impairment in nerves or muscles in the past 6 months?	YES ☐ NO ☐

10.   Do you have any other medical condition not listed above or do you have two or more medical conditions?

If you have other medical conditions, answer questions 10a-10c   If **NO** ☐ read the Page 4 recommendations

10a.	Have you experienced a blackout, fainted, or lost consciousness as a result of a head injury within the last 12 months **OR** have you had a diagnosed concussion within the last 12 months?	YES ☐ NO ☐
10b.	Do you have a medical condition that is not listed (such as epilepsy, neurological conditions, kidney problems)?	YES ☐ NO ☐
10c.	Do you currently live with two or more medical conditions?	YES ☐ NO ☐

PLEASE LIST YOUR MEDICAL CONDITION(S) AND ANY RELATED MEDICATIONS HERE: _____

_____

GO to Page 4 for recommendations about your current medical condition(s) and sign the PARTICIPANT DECLARATION.

FIGURE 5.1   *(continued)*

Reprinted with permission from the PAR-Q+ Collaboration and the authors of the PAR-Q+ (Dr. Darren Warburton, Dr. Norman Gledhill, Dr. Veronica Jamnik, and Dr. Shannon Bredin).

2020 PAR-Q+

If you answered NO to all of the FOLLOW-UP questions (pgs. 2-3) about your medical condition, you are ready to become more physically active - sign the PARTICIPANT DECLARATION below:

▶ It is advised that you consult a qualified exercise professional to help you develop a safe and effective physical activity plan to meet your health needs.

▶ You are encouraged to start slowly and build up gradually - 20 to 60 minutes of low to moderate intensity exercise, 3-5 days per week including aerobic and muscle strengthening exercises.

▶ As you progress, you should aim to accumulate 150 minutes or more of moderate intensity physical activity per week.

▶ If you are over the age of 45 yr and **NOT** accustomed to regular vigorous to maximal effort exercise, consult a qualified exercise professional before engaging in this intensity of exercise.

If you answered YES to one or more of the follow-up questions about your medical condition:
You should seek further information before becoming more physically active or engaging in a fitness appraisal. You should complete the specially designed online screening and exercise recommendations program - the **ePARmed-X+ at www.eparmedx.com** and/or visit a qualified exercise professional to work through the ePARmed-X+ and for further information.

⚠ **Delay becoming more active if:**

You have a temporary illness such as a cold or fever; it is best to wait until you feel better.

You are pregnant - talk to your health care practitioner, your physician, a qualified exercise professional, and/or complete the ePARmed-X+ **at www.eparmedx.com** before becoming more physically active.

Your health changes - talk to your doctor or qualified exercise professional before continuing with any physical activity program.

● You are encouraged to photocopy the PAR-Q+. You must use the entire questionnaire and NO changes are permitted.
● The authors, the PAR-Q+ Collaboration, partner organizations, and their agents assume no liability for persons who undertake physical activity and/or make use of the PAR-Q+ or ePARmed-X+. If in doubt after completing the questionnaire, consult your doctor prior to physical activity.

PARTICIPANT DECLARATION

● All persons who have completed the PAR-Q+ please read and sign the declaration below.

● If you are less than the legal age required for consent or require the assent of a care provider, your parent, guardian or care provider must also sign this form.

I, the undersigned, have read, understood to my full satisfaction and completed this questionnaire. I acknowledge that this physical activity clearance is valid for a maximum of 12 months from the date it is completed and becomes invalid if my condition changes. I also acknowledge that the community/fitness center may retain a copy of this form for records. In these instances, it will maintain the confidentiality of the same, complying with applicable law.

NAME _____   DATE _____

SIGNATURE _____   WITNESS _____

SIGNATURE OF PARENT/GUARDIAN/CARE PROVIDER _____

———— For more information, please contact ————
www.eparmedx.com
Email: eparmedx@gmail.com

Citation for PAR-Q+
Warburton DER, Jamnik VK, Bredin SSD, and Gledhill N on behalf of the PAR-Q+ Collaboration. The Physical Activity Readiness Questionnaire for Everyone (PAR-Q+) and Electronic Physical Activity Readiness Medical Examination (ePARmed-X+). Health & Fitness Journal of Canada 4(2):3-23, 2011.

The PAR-Q+ was created using the evidence-based AGREE process (1) by the PAR-Q+ Collaboration chaired by Dr. Darren E. R. Warburton with Dr. Norman Gledhill, Dr. Veronica Jamnik, and Dr. Donald C. McKenzie (2). Production of this document has been made possible through financial contributions from the Public Health Agency of Canada and the BC Ministry of Health Services. The views expressed herein do not necessarily represent the views of the Public Health Agency of Canada or the BC Ministry of Health Services.

Key References
1. Jamnik VK, Warburton DER, Makarski J, McKenzie DC, Shephard RJ, Stone J, and Gledhill N. Enhancing the effectiveness of clearance for physical activity participation; background and overall process. APNM 36(S1):S3-S13, 2011.
2. Warburton DER, Gledhill N, Jamnik VK, Bredin SSD, McKenzie DC, Stone J, Charlesworth S, and Shephard RJ. Evidence-based risk assessment and recommendations for physical activity clearance; Consensus Document. APNM 36(S1):S266-s298, 2011.
3. Chisholm DM, Collis ML, Kulak LL, Davenport W, and Gruber N. Physical activity readiness. British Columbia Medical Journal. 1975;17:375-378.
4. Thomas S, Reading J, and Shephard RJ. Revision of the Physical Activity Readiness Questionnaire (PAR-Q). Canadian Journal of Sport Science 1992;17:4 338-345.

FIGURE 5.1 (continued)

Reprinted with permission from the PAR-Q+ Collaboration and the authors of the PAR-Q+ (Dr. Darren Warburton, Dr. Norman Gledhill, Dr. Veronica Jamnik, and Dr. Shannon Bredin).

Heart Rate Assessment

The purpose of this test is to assess resting heart rate (RHR). You will need a stopwatch or timer. True RHR is measured just before the client gets out of bed in the morning (without being startled by an alarm). However, this test will give you a reasonable idea about the person's health and fitness, with fitter individuals having a lower RHR. Note that heart rate (HR) changes by 7 to 15 beats per minute (BPM) when individuals transition from lying to standing due to the effects of gravity and the actions of the postural muscles. Therefore, it is important to consider the position in which you measure the RHR. The client should be seated quietly for at least five minutes before you start to measure RHR. Place the fingertips on a pulse site. Use the following steps to complete a RHR assessment:

1. Place the tips of your index and middle fingers (not the thumb, which will measure your own pulse) over the artery and lightly apply pressure. Commonly used sites to measure RHR are the radial pulse, which is palpated with two fingers on the wrist at the base of the thumb (see figure 5.2a), or the carotid pulse, which is palpated by placing the fingertips on the neck, just beside the larynx (see figure 5.2b). Heavy pressure should be avoided because the carotid arteries contain baroreceptors that sense increases in pressure and respond by slowing the HR.

2. To determine RHR, count the number of beats for 30 seconds and then multiply by two to determine beats per minute (BPM).

3. Because you are counting cardiac cycles, the first pulse measured should commence with the number 0.

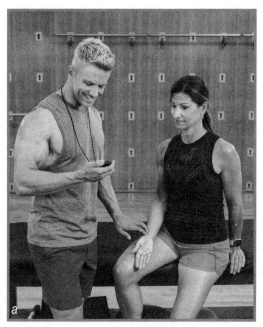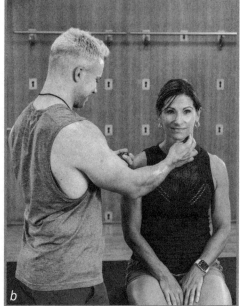

FIGURE 5.2   Pulse sites: *(a)* radial and *(b)* carotid.

Resting Blood Pressure Assessment

Blood pressure is reasonably simple to test but may take a little practice. The measurement of resting blood pressure is an integral component of the pre-exercise evaluation (ACSM, 2017). High blood pressure is a silent disease that affects millions of adults. In the period between 2017 and 2018, the prevalence of age-adjusted hypertension was 45.4% among adults and was higher among men (52.0%) than women (39.7%) (Ostchega et al., 2020). Knowing a client's blood pressure can allow you to refer them to a medical practitioner if necessary, especially if the client is unaware of their condition.

Before the test, make sure your blood pressure cuff is accurate and the size is correct (the bladder within the cuff should encircle at least 80 percent of the upper arm). Many adults require a larger cuff. Before the reading, your client should have no food or drink for 30 minutes beforehand and should empty their bladder. In a quiet environment, ideally, have your client sit with back support and both feet on the floor with their arms supported at heart level, but if back support is not available, you can ask your client to sit upright on a bench. Allow them to sit quietly for at least five minutes, then follow these steps:

1. Wrap the cuff firmly against bare skin on the upper arm at heart level, aligning the cuff with the brachial artery (see figure 5.3a).

2. Place the stethoscope chest piece over the brachial artery (see figure 5.3b).

3. Quickly inflate the cuff pressure (it should be 20 mm Hg above the first "beat" you hear, called a Korotkoff sound).

4. Slowly release pressure.

5. To measure blood pressure, note the systolic blood pressure (SBP) at the point at which the first two or more Korotkoff sounds can be heard and the diastolic blood pressure (DBP) at the point before Korotkoff sounds can no longer be heard.

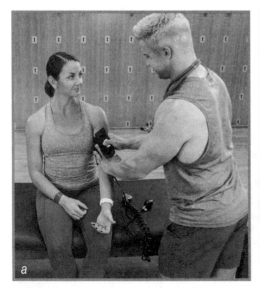 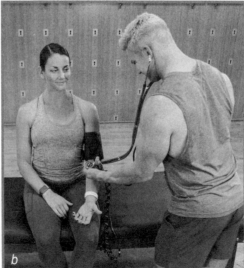

FIGURE 5.3   Blood pressure reading: (a) align cuff with brachial artery and (b) place stethoscope over brachial artery.

Joint Flexibility and Muscle Length Assessment

The Thomas test for hip flexion and quadriceps length assesses a critical area. Due to the origin and insertion of the iliopsoas, or inner hip muscles (from T12 along the anterior border of the spine and lumbar discs to the upper femur), tightness in this area of the body can cause excessive lumbar curvature (known as *lordosis*), often leading to lower back pain. The vital information gained from this test will assist in knowing what areas of the body would benefit from a focused flexibility program and may even help prevent lower back pain. This test should not be performed on clients suffering from lower back pain unless cleared by their physician.

To perform the assessment you will need a sturdy table. First, briefly explain the purpose of the test and provide a brief demonstration. After some light warm-up and stretching, instruct your client to sit at the end of a table with their mid-thigh aligned with the table edge and follow these steps:

1. Have your client lift both knees gently toward their chest and slowly assist them to roll back onto the table, supine, back and shoulders down. Their lower back and sacrum should be completely flat on the table (see figure 5.4a).

2. Instruct your client to pull one leg deeper towards their chest by reaching with both hands to grasp the backside of the thigh, without raising the torso from the table.

3. Have them slowly lower the other leg, allowing the thigh to move towards the table, bringing this hip into extension (the lowered leg side) and thereby stretching the hip flexors. You can assist your client in reaching this position by holding the lifted leg in place. (see figure 5.4b).

To interpret the test, the back of the lower thigh should touch the table, the knee should demonstrate 80 degrees of flexion, and the knee should remain aligned straight and should not externally rotate. If the sacrum is flat, the lower leg does not touch the table, and the knee is extended beyond 80 degrees, then there is a great likelihood of tightness in the iliopsoas and rectus femoris. If the back of the knee does not touch the table, but the knee does flex to 80 degrees, then it may be the psoas but not the rectus femoris. If the back of the lower leg does touch the table, but the knee does not flex to 80 degrees, then it's more likely to be tightness in the rectus femoris.

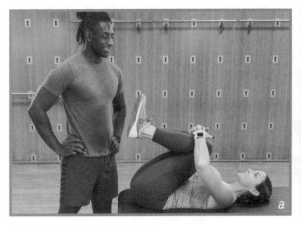 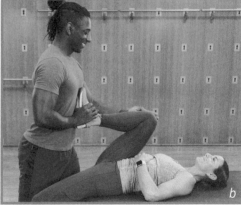

FIGURE 5.4   Thomas test.

Muscular Endurance Assessments

There are multiple tests to assess muscular endurance. According to Stuart McGill, PhD, an expert in spine function and author of a book on the prevention and rehabilitation of low back disorders, "strength appears to have little, or a very weak, relationship with low back health. Muscle endurance, when separated from strength, appears to be linked with better back health" (2015). This is especially true for the side-bridge endurance test (described later in the chapter). Although this test is not a primary indicator of current or future back problems, it can indicate a lack of torso stability.

Aside from back health, assessing muscular endurance through the following tests provides information about the level at which your group should begin. Muscular endurance movements are foundational to strength training. If your clients lack muscular endurance, they should be using more body weight or light load movements to build the prerequisite type of fitness.

Push-Up Test

The push-up test is simple to perform; all that is needed is a mat and a small rolled-up towel. It provides a good indication of upper-body muscular endurance, specifically the "pushing" muscles—the pectoralis, the triceps, and the anterior deltoids. Because strength can vary greatly between men and women, the test can be performed in a modified position for women or deconditioned individuals. The test may not be appropriate for clients with wrist, elbow, or shoulder problems.

Explain the purpose of the test and demonstrate the correct push-up technique, making sure the client understands fully. Warm up and stretch as necessary. The hands should be positioned shoulder-width apart, directly below the shoulders, and face forward. Hips and shoulders should be aligned and the torso should remain rigid, like a plank. The knees can be off the ground as in a standard push-up or on the ground for a modified push-up. The goal of the test is for the client to perform as many complete and consecutive push-ups as possible before reaching the point of fatigue. Make sure your clients understand that there should be no rest between the repetitions and only correctly performed push-ups are counted. Perform the test as follows:

1. The test starts in the "down" position, with the chest resting on a small rolled-up towel, elbows bent and body lowered (see figure 5.5a). The client can start at any time.
2. Count each complete repetition. A full repetition is described as full elbow extension with the spine completely rigid and straight at the top of the movement (see figure 5.5b), then lowered back to the down position with the chest touching the towel without the stomach or body resting on the mat.
3. The test is finished when the client is unable to complete another repetition or fails to maintain correct technique.
4. The score should be recorded to compare to the later retest. It can also be used to compare to normative data for the same age or gender group.

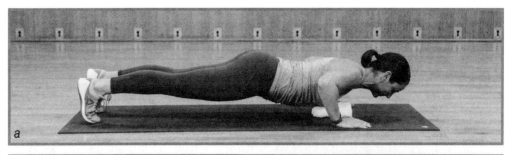

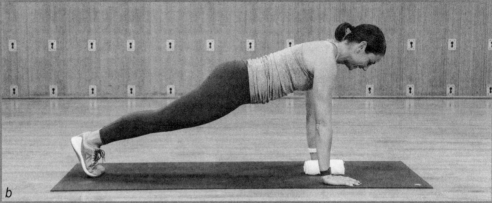

FIGURE 5.5   Push-up test.

The push-up test can also easily be performed in a group setting. Simply have your group start the assessment together and count their own repetitions. Clients who would prefer for their results to be confidential can simply note their results on a sheet; this way progress can be easily measured several weeks later. For more well-conditioned individuals, splitting clients into pairs and having them count reps for each other is a fun way to create some healthy competition.

Bodyweight Squat Test

The bodyweight squat test is useful to assess lower-extremity muscular endurance. This test is only suitable for individuals who can perform a squat with correct technique. It should not be utilized for clients with knee issues or balance concerns or for frail individuals with lower-extremity weakness.

Explain the purpose of the test and demonstrate correct technique, making sure the client understands fully. Warm up and stretch as necessary. The depth of the squat should ideally be parallel to the floor. If the client cannot squat to that depth, make a note of it on the testing form to allow a comparison for further testing. The client may extend their arms in front of their body to assist balance. The goal of the test is to perform as many correct repetitions as possible. Allow the client a few practice repetitions to ascertain the correct depth and technique, then start when ready. Perform the test as follows:

1. The client starts in an upright stance with hips fully extended and knees straight but not locked. Arms are resting beside the body, eyes forward, shoulders back and down (see figure 5.6*a*).

2. Count only correctly performed repetitions. This means they should lower as far as possible, ideally to parallel to the floor (see figure 5.6b), and back to a fully upright stance.

3. When the client can no longer perform the squats to the correct depth, pauses to rest, or demonstrates poor form, the test is terminated.

4. The score should be recorded to compare to the later retest. It can also be used to compare to normative data for the same age or gender group.

The bodyweight squat assessment is another good one to perform as a group. Again, individuals may either count and record their own reps or work with a partner.

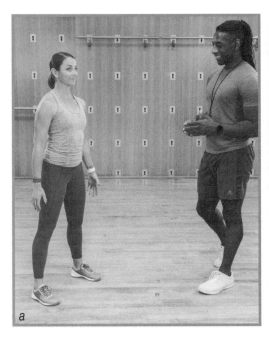
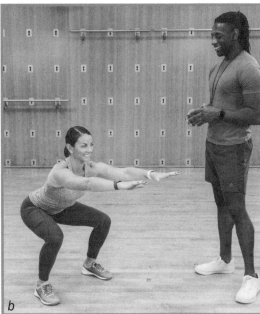

FIGURE 5.6   Bodyweight squat test.

Cardiorespiratory Assessments

Cardiorespiratory fitness (CRF) is related to the ability to sustain dynamic, moderate- to vigorous-intensity exercise of large muscle groups for prolonged periods of time. Performance of exercise at this level of physical exertion depends on the integrated physiologic and functional state of the respiratory, cardiovascular, and musculoskeletal systems (Blair et al., 1995). It is considered an important health-related component to physical fitness because low levels of performance have been linked to increased risk of premature death from cardiovascular disease. Because increases in CRF are associated with a decrease in death from all causes, it is an important assessment to include, both for health reasons and to establish a baseline of fitness for future retests.

Because many cardiorespiratory tests require specific equipment, some guidelines should be noted. If the client is deconditioned but able to walk, the Rockport walking test is a good option. For a runner, then a graded treadmill test or a 1.5-mile run (used for U.S. Navy personnel) would be preferable. The YMCA step test is another popular assessment and needs only a 12-inch (30.5 cm) step, a stopwatch or timer, and a metronome (a BPM timer). The step test, however, is not appropriate for individuals with knee issues. If assessing a cyclist, then either a field test time trial or the Astrand-Rhyming cycle ergometer test is best. No matter how you decide to assess for CRF, keep it specific to the individual and their needs, exercise history, and physical limitations.

Jumping Jack Test

If assessing cardiorespiratory fitness in a group session, then a jumping jack test is a simple method. This test is most appropriate to individuals who can jump; however, if jumping is contraindicated (for example, because of knee problems) then a modified, low-impact variation can be performed. Perform the test as follows:

1. Measure resting HR before the test and record BPM. Recording pretest HR provides a baseline to compare to the recovery HR posttest.
2. Perform one minute of jumping jacks, with full range of motion and arms fully extended, touching overhead.
3. Measure HR for 10 to 15 seconds immediately following exercise and record the number in BPM.
4. One minute later, measure HR for 30 to 60 seconds and record in BPM.
5. Subtract the recovery BPM from the working BPM. Because a more conditioned individual's heart rate drops faster than a less fit person's, a higher number indicates a greater level of fitness.

YMCA Step Test

Another cardiorespiratory test that works well in group settings is the YMCA step test. This assessment is ideal for low-risk, apparently healthy, nonathletic individuals between the ages of 20 and 59. It is not recommended with individuals with knee pain or knee injuries. You will need a 12-inch (30.5 cm) step, stopwatch, and a metronome (you can download one as an app on a phone) set to 96 clicks per minute, which represents 24 step cycles per minute.

Before you begin, you should describe and demonstrate the four-part stepping motion ("up, up, down, down"), noting that either foot may lead the step sequence. Provide a short practice to allow clients to familiarize themselves with the step speed. The goal of the test is to step up and down on the 12-inch riser for three minutes. Immediately after the test, measure the client's heart rate for one full minute. It is important to have the client sit down and remain quiet following the test to allow the trainer to accurately assess heart rate. Perform the test as follows:

1. The client begins stepping on the trainer's cue, then the stopwatch is started.
2. Coach the initial steps to ensure the correct pace is being maintained with the metronome. Motivate for the remaining time for the client to stay on task.
3. At the three-minute mark, the test is stopped and the client immediately sits down.
4. Measure the client's HR for a full minute. It is essential to begin the heart rate check within five seconds of the completion of the test. Because immediate postexercise heart rate should decrease over the minute, a lower score is ideal.
5. Classify the client's score using the data in figure 5.7 for men and women, then record the values.

After recording the results of your cardiorespiratory assessments, have your client complete a three- to five-minute cool-down followed by some lower-limb stretching. Observe the client for any negative symptoms that may arise, such as dizziness or accelerated heart rate. If any other signs or symptoms arise during the exercise testing, the client's personal physician should be notified immediately. Emergency medical services should be called if severe signs or symptoms arise, such as unconsciousness, chest pains, or any other signs or symptoms of cardiac distress or extreme difficulty in breathing that is not controlled by rest.

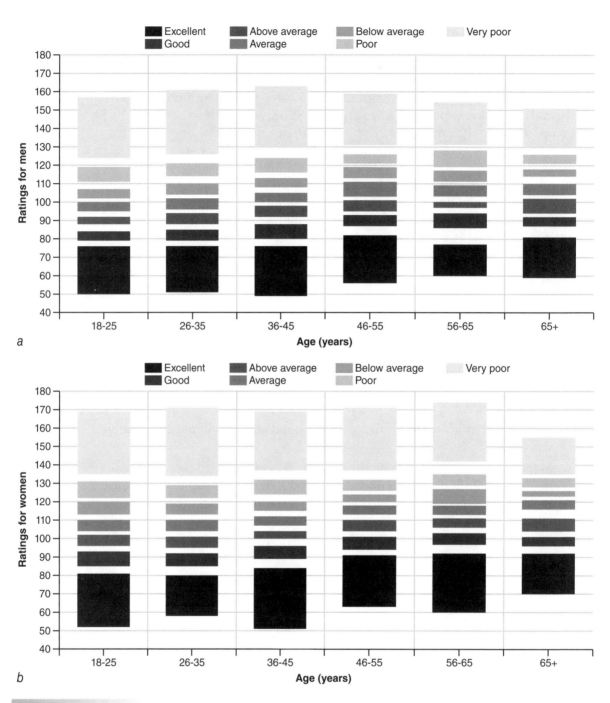

FIGURE 5.7   YMCA step test norms for *(a)* men and *(b)* women.

Data from *YMCA Fitness Testing and Assessment Manual*, 4th ed. (Champaign, IL: Human Kinetics, 2000).

Body Composition Assessments

Anthropometric measurements such as body mass index (BMI) can be simple to assess. There are many methods to measure body composition, including sophisticated machines such as air displacement plethysmography, hydrostatic weighing, and dual-energy X-ray absorptiometry (DEXA). However, these are not only complex, but financially and logistically out of reach for most small businesses and trainers. The simplest and most affordable options are skinfold calipers or a tape measure.

Note that it is advisable to perform all anthropometric measurements in a one-on-one setting. These types of tests can be very intimidating and stressful for certain individuals. These tests can be offered as add-ons for a small fee and can be extremely helpful in helping motivate your clients. Additionally, tests and retests can set the stage for referrals. Once clients see concrete improvements, whether weight loss or improved strength and conditioning, it's a surefire way to demonstrate the value of your program.

BMI

Body mass index (BMI) can be a useful measurement, but because calculations do not take into account body composition (amount of lean muscle mass versus fat mass), it is not useful for all populations. Muscle tissue is extremely dense and significantly heavier than fat mass, so a lean, muscular individual can score badly on a BMI test, especially if they're not very tall. Therefore, only use BMI testing on more deconditioned or sedentary clients and not on muscular individuals, for whom results can be skewed. The calculation can be compared to norms and help you set realistic and motivating goals. Although there are formulas available to calculate BMI, you can use figure 5.8 to determine your client's BMI classification using only their weight and height.

Circumference Measurements

Perhaps the most meaningful measurement from a client's point of view is circumference or girth, which can be particularly helpful when clients are gaining muscle. The scale can move in the wrong direction for weight-loss clients who are gaining lean muscle mass, leading to confusion and frustration, but the scale combined with a tape measure can be quite powerful. When inches are lost and weight is gained, then body composition has clearly changed for the better! With some simple explanations it's easy for clients to see they are making progress.

WAIST-TO-HIP RATIO (WHR)

There is a strong correlation between excess abdominal (visceral) fat and a number of health risks, including type 2 diabetes, hypertension, and hypercholesterolemia (ACE, 2014). This means that location of body fat deposits is important in assessing disease risk. Apple-shaped (android) persons retain

	Normal						Overweight					Obese						
BMI	19	20	21	22	23	24	25	26	27	28	29	30	31	32	33	34	35	
Height (inches)									Body weight (pounds)									
58	91	96	100	105	110	115	119	124	129	134	138	143	148	153	158	162	167	
59	94	99	104	109	114	119	124	128	133	138	143	148	153	158	163	168	173	
60	97	102	107	112	118	123	128	133	138	143	148	153	158	163	168	174	179	
61	100	106	111	116	122	127	132	137	143	148	153	158	164	169	174	180	185	
62	104	109	115	120	126	131	136	142	147	153	158	164	169	175	180	186	191	
63	107	113	118	124	130	135	141	146	152	158	163	169	175	180	186	191	197	
64	110	116	122	128	134	140	145	151	157	163	169	174	180	186	192	197	204	
65	114	120	126	132	138	144	150	156	162	168	174	180	186	192	198	204	210	
66	118	124	130	136	142	148	155	161	167	173	179	186	192	198	204	210	216	
67	121	127	134	140	146	153	159	166	172	178	185	191	198	204	211	217	223	
68	125	131	138	144	151	158	164	171	177	184	190	197	203	210	216	223	230	
69	128	135	143	149	155	162	169	176	182	189	196	203	209	216	223	230	236	
70	132	139	146	153	160	167	174	181	188	195	202	209	216	222	229	236	243	
71	136	143	150	157	165	172	179	186	193	200	208	215	222	229	236	243	250	
72	140	147	154	162	169	177	184	191	199	206	213	221	228	235	242	250	258	
73	144	151	159	166	174	182	189	197	204	212	219	227	235	242	250	257	265	
74	148	155	163	171	179	186	194	202	210	218	225	233	241	249	256	264	272	
75	152	160	168	176	184	192	200	208	216	224	232	240	248	256	264	272	279	
76	156	164	172	180	189	197	205	213	221	230	238	246	254	263	271	279	287	

FIGURE 5.8 Body mass index (BMI) calculator.

Reprinted by permission from ACSM, *ACSM's Complete Guide to Fitness & Health*, 2nd ed., edited by B. Brushman (Champaign, IL: Human Kinetics, 2017), 352; Adapted from U.S. Department of Health and Human Services, National Heart, Lung, and Blood Institute, 1998, *Clinical Guidelines on the Identification, Evaluation, and Treatment of Overweight and Obesity in Adults: The Evidence Report.* http://www.nhlbi.nih.gov/health/educational/lose_wt/BMI/bmi_tbl.pdf

body fat around the midsection, whereas pear-shaped (gynoid) individuals hold theirs around their hips and thighs. A simple and effective assessment is to calculate the waist-to-hip ratio by measuring both the waist and hips (either in inches or centimeters) and dividing the waist measurement by the hip measurement. You can compare your client's results with the data in table 5.1 to assess their level of risk. If your client's result is excellent or good, they would

TABLE 5.1 Waist-to-Hip Ratio Norms

Gender	Excellent	Good	Average	Poor
Male	<0.85	0.85-0.89	0.90-0.95	≥0.95
Female	<0.75	0.75-0.79	0.80-0.86	≥0.86

Data from ACSM Guidelines for Exercise Prescription (2018); Data from G.A. Bray and D.S. Gray, "Obesity, Part I, Pathogenesis," *Western Journal of Medicine* 149 (1988): 429-41.

				Extreme obesity														
36	37	38	39	40	41	42	43	44	45	46	47	48	49	50	51	52	53	54
172	177	181	186	191	196	201	205	210	215	220	224	229	234	239	244	248	253	258
178	183	188	193	198	203	208	212	217	222	227	232	237	242	247	252	257	262	267
184	189	194	199	204	209	215	220	225	230	235	240	245	250	255	261	266	271	276
190	195	201	206	211	217	222	227	232	238	243	248	254	259	264	269	275	280	285
196	202	207	213	218	224	229	235	240	248	251	256	262	267	273	278	284	289	295
203	208	216	220	225	231	237	242	248	254	259	265	270	278	282	287	293	299	304
209	215	221	227	232	238	244	250	256	262	267	273	279	285	291	296	302	308	314
216	222	228	234	240	246	252	258	264	270	276	282	288	294	300	306	312	318	324
223	229	235	241	247	253	260	266	272	278	284	291	297	303	309	315	322	328	334
230	236	242	249	255	261	268	274	280	287	293	299	306	312	319	325	331	338	344
236	243	249	256	262	269	276	282	289	295	302	308	315	322	328	335	341	348	354
243	250	257	263	270	277	285	291	297	304	311	318	324	331	338	345	351	358	365
250	259	264	271	278	285	292	299	306	313	320	327	334	341	348	355	362	369	376
257	265	272	279	286	293	301	308	315	322	329	338	343	351	358	365	372	379	386
265	272	279	287	294	302	309	316	324	331	338	346	353	361	368	375	383	390	397
273	280	288	295	302	310	318	325	333	340	348	355	363	371	378	386	393	401	408
280	287	295	303	311	319	326	334	342	350	358	365	373	381	389	396	404	412	420
287	295	303	311	319	327	335	343	351	359	367	375	383	391	399	407	415	423	431
295	304	312	320	328	336	344	353	361	369	377	385	394	402	410	418	426	435	443

be classified as low risk for cardiovascular and metabolic diseases. Average or poor classifications would indicate the need for weight loss and increased physical activity and improved cardiovascular fitness.

WAIST CIRCUMFERENCE

Because waist circumference correlates with so many health risks, a waistline measurement is a simple but effective assessment. Waist circumference may be a superior measure to BMI for this purpose. Although BMI and waist circumference are correlated, waist circumference is a better measure of visceral adiposity, which can vary within a given BMI (Despres, 2012). Perform the test as follows:

1. The measurement should be taken with your client in a standing position.
2. A horizontal measurement is taken at the height of the iliac crest, usually at the level of the navel (see figure 5.9). The tape should be placed on the skin surface without compressing the subcutaneous adipose tissue. All measures should be made with a flexible but inelastic tape measure.
3. Once you've taken the measurements, compare the numbers to norms in figure 5.10 (Bray, 2004).

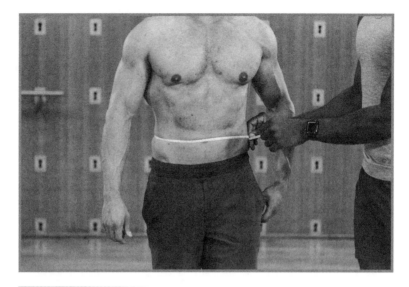

FIGURE 5.9   Waist circumference measurement.

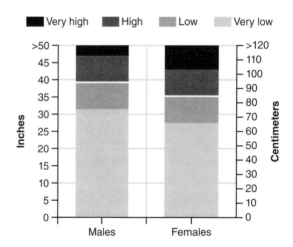

FIGURE 5.10   Waist circumference norms in adults.

Data from Bray (2004).

SKINFOLD TESTING

Body fat can be either subcutaneous or visceral. Subcutaneous fat is located between the skin and muscle, whereas visceral fat sits below the muscle in the abdomen and surrounds the organs. It is assumed that approximately one-third of total fat is subcutaneous (Lohman, 1981).

Subcutaneous fat can be measured with a device called a skinfold caliper. The accuracy of this testing relies on the skill of the practitioner. Perform the test as follows:

1. All measurements should be made on the right side of the body with the client standing upright. The three sites for men are the pectoral, thigh, and abdomen. For women, measure the triceps, suprailiac, and thigh.

2. The caliper should be held one centimeter away from the thumb and finger and placed directly on bare skin, perpendicular to the skinfold, halfway between the crest and base of the fold.

3. The pinch should be held for one to two seconds and maintained while reading the caliper.

4. Take duplicate measurements at each site and retest if results are not within one to two millimeters of one another. Rotate through measurement sites or allow time for skin to regain normal texture and thickness. Following are standardized descriptions of skinfold measurement sites (see figure 5.11):

   - *Abdominals (men)*: measurement is taken next to the navel.
   - *Triceps (women)*: measurement is taken along the back of the upper arm.
   - *Pectoral (men)*: measurement is taken between the armpit and nipple.
   - *Suprailiac (women)*: measurement is taken just above the iliac crest.
   - *Thigh (men and women)*: measurement is taken in the middle of the upper thigh.

Body fat percentage can be calculated with the right tools and formulas, but if the trainer is inexperienced or uses poor technique, the margin of error can be as great as 6 to 8 percent. When comparing caliper methods with hydrostatic weighing (considered the benchmark for measuring body composition), there can be a 2.0 to 3.5 percent difference in the results. Unfortunately, hydrostatic weighing is expensive, time consuming, and requires substantial space and a high level of expertise. Furthermore, the process involves being completely submerged underwater with all air exhaled from the lungs, which may be an uncomfortable proposition for some clients. This makes testing with skinfold calipers a good option. If you decide to use skinfold measurements, make sure you have plenty of practice before using this method with clients.

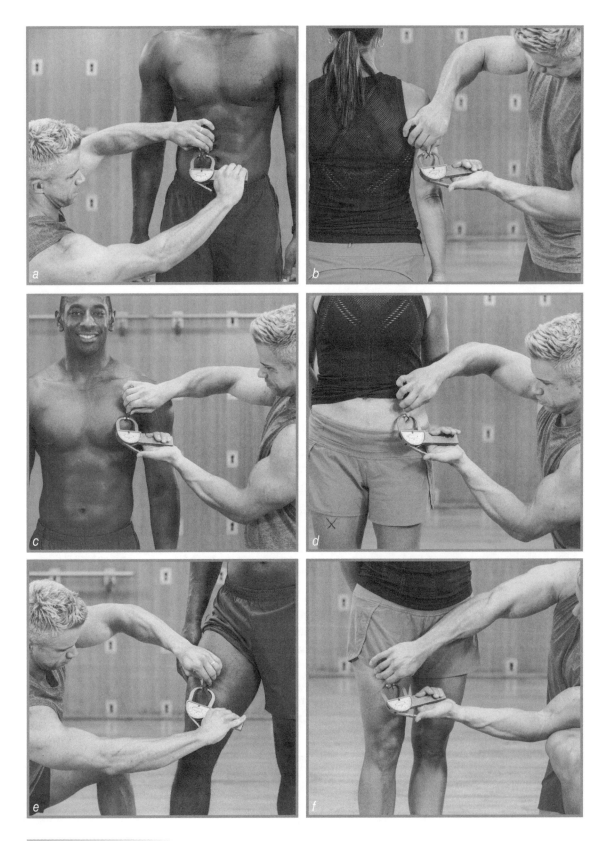

FIGURE 5.11 Skinfold measurement sites: *(a)* abdominals for men, *(b)* triceps for women, *(c)* pectoral for men, *(d)* suprailiac for women, *(e)* thigh for men, and *(f)* thigh for women.

Balance Assessment

Balance is another important function to assess. Balance training may decrease the likelihood of falling, so setting a baseline can be helpful in monitoring progress. Assessing balance is an especially good idea if you work with older adults, for whom a fall can be deadly. Because balance is so critical to daily function, yet may seem a little nebulous to measure, a formal assessment like the stork-stand test works well.

Before you begin, you will need an open area with a flat, nonslip surface and a stopwatch. Clearly explain the purpose of the test and ask the client to remove their shoes (ideally, shoes would not be worn). You can allow approximately one minute of practice trials. Perform the test as follows:

1. Instruct the client to stand with feet together and hands on hips.
2. Instruct the client to raise one foot off the ground and bring that foot to lightly touch the inside of the stance leg, just below the knee (see figure 5.12*a*).
3. The client then raises the heel of the stance foot off the floor and balances on the ball of the foot (see figure 5.12*b*), keeping their eyes open the entire time. Begin timing.
4. The timing stops with any loss of balance or when any of the following occurs: (1) the hand(s) come off the hips; (2) the stance or supporting foot inverts, everts, or moves in any direction; (3) any part of the elevated foot loses contact with the stance leg; or (4) the heel of the stance leg touches the floor.

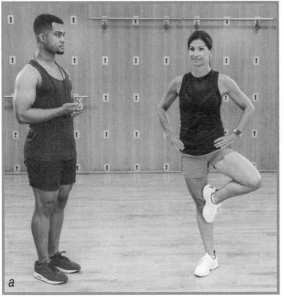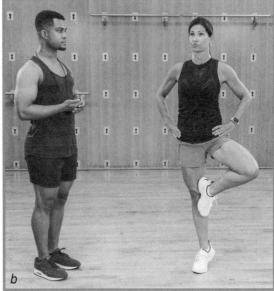

FIGURE 5.12   Stork-stand test.

5. Norms for the test are provided in table 5.2. Should your client score average to poor, balance work would be advisable.

TABLE 5.2   Stork-Stand Test Norms

Rating	Excellent	Good	Average	Fair	Poor
Males	>50 seconds	41-50 seconds	31-40 seconds	20-30 seconds	<20 seconds
Females	>30 seconds	25-30 seconds	16-24 seconds	10-15 seconds	<10 seconds

Reprinted from B.L. Johnson and J.K. Nelson, *Practical Measurements for Evaluation in Physical Education*, 4th ed. (Minneapolis, MN: Burgess, 1986).

Core Function Assessments

Assessing core function can be very involved or reasonably simple. For your purposes, the plank test or side-bridge endurance test are good places to start when assessing the muscular endurance of the core. Both tests provide beneficial information that in turn can direct your program design. The plank requires reasonable amounts of trunk stability, which is the ability of the core musculature to sustain a contraction without the loss of position or body control. This ability may reduce the likelihood of low back pain. The side-bridge endurance test assesses endurance of the lateral core musculature (transverse abdominis, obliques, quadratus lumborum, and erector spinae). This test requires greater shoulder strength and stability, so if your client has shoulder issues, the prone plank may be a better choice.

Plank Test

You will need a mat and a stopwatch for this test. Before you begin, clearly explain the purpose of the plank test and both describe and demonstrate correct body alignment. Allow the client some practice trials. Contraindications to these tests include shoulder pain or injury, acute back pain or spasms, or a recent back surgery. Should deficiencies present during this test, a diligent core training program should be included in training sessions. When the client is ready, perform the test as follows:

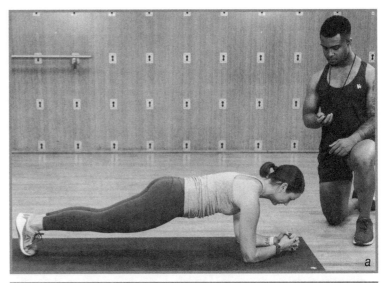

1. Instruct the client to assume a forearm plank position, elbows bent and directly under the shoulders with the spine in a neutral alignment. The legs can either be fully extended (see figure 5.13a) or in a modified position on the knees (see figure 5.13b).

2. Start the stopwatch the moment the client assumes the position. The goal is to hold the position for as long as possible, with good technique.

3. Terminate the test when there is a noticeable change in torso position or the client voluntarily stops, then record the client's time.

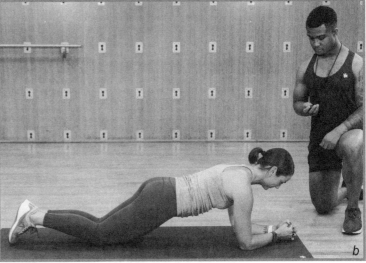

FIGURE 5.13   Plank test: *(a)* full and *(b)* modified.

Side-Bridge Endurance Test

This timed test involves static, isometric contractions of the trunk that stabilize the spine. It is an excellent test to assess this element of spinal stabilization. The test should not be performed by those with shoulder pain or weakness, who suffer from lower back pain, or who have had a recent back surgery.

Before you begin, you will need a stopwatch and mat. Clearly explain the purpose of the test, describing correct body position. When the client is ready, perform the test as follows:

1. The client assumes a position on their side with the elbow under the shoulder and the upper arm directly in front of the body with the palm of the hand facing downwards for balance and support. The other arm is resting along the body.

2. Instruct the client to lift the hips up to assume a full side-bridge position, maintaining both legs in a fully extended stance (see figure 5.14a) with the sides of the feet on the floor in a tandem toe-to-heel position. When the hips are elevated off the mat, the head, neck, torso, hips, and legs should all be aligned.

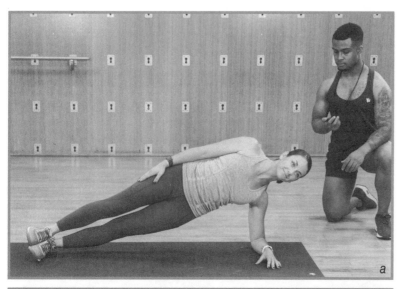

3. The client attempts to maintain this aligned position for as long as possible. Once the client breaks the position (lowers the hips) and there is a noticeable deviation in trunk position or the hips shift forward or backwards, the test is terminated.

4. Record the client's time on the testing form and position then repeat on the other side and record the values for future retests.

Both plank and side-bridge assessments can be performed in a small-group setting at the beginning stages of a closed session. You can start the timer and call out time every 5 to 10 seconds so clients can monitor how long they've been holding their planks. Working with a partner for this particular test is a good idea so the observer can keep an eye on the quality of the plank.

FIGURE 5.14   Side-bridge endurance test: *(a)* full and *(b)* modified.

Skill-Related Assessment

Testing for skill-related ability should be very specific to the needs and goals of the client. These types of assessments are helpful when the client is involved in sports such as tennis, soccer, football, or basketball. These sports involve rapid changes of direction and a high demand for agility, acceleration, and deceleration and have specific fitness and training requirements. This makes an assessment important for establishing a baseline for further retests.

Agility, or the ability to change direction rapidly without the loss of body control, can be trained and improved. Speed and agility tests can be useful to predict the client's athletic potential and help motivate them to set competitive goals outside of the gym setting. Sports performance testing is only recommended or necessary for those individuals who are well conditioned and pursuing the types of sports that demand these abilities. The Pro Agility Test, also known as the 20-yard agility test or the 5-10-5 shuttle run, is used by both the NFL and the U.S. Women's Soccer Team, along with a battery of other assessments.

Other performance-based tests are the standing long jump test, the vertical jump test, and the 40-yard dash. All these tests and the Pro Agility Test allow you to make comparisons to normative data. You can also come up with your own simple tests, such as a shuttle run performed with a variety of footwork (e.g., a carioca, lateral shuffle, or forward running and back pedaling). Set up two cones, 5 to 10 yards apart, and have the client go back and forth using a given footwork pattern as many times as possible in 30 seconds. This type of test can even be used in a group setting by having one partner time while the other performs the test, then swapping.

In the Trenches

Luis Castaneda, an employee of the YMCA in Santa Clarita, California, takes a very simple approach when it comes to assessments. Luis works mostly with clients aged 50 and older. They all fill out an HRA form and signed consent form. He likes to interview his clients to get a background on what they do, what they want, and if there's anything he needs to know specifically about their health, such as knee or back issues. He then has them walk on a treadmill to gauge their cardiovascular fitness with a talk test. However, he doesn't tell them it's an assessment, finding that he gets a more accurate result when clients don't know it's a test and subsequently try too hard.

Andy Leskin, of the Gaims Fitness Company in the San Fernando Valley, California, takes a reasonably detailed approach with his SGT business. His facility caters to those over age 50, with the average age being closer to mid-60s and some even in their late 80s. Clients are presented with a package including informed consent, liability waiver, PAR-Q+, emergency contact, physician information, and a physician's release, if indicated by the PAR-Q+. Being a boutique facility, assessment is included in the cost of the sessions. If fitness tests are not performed, clients may be recommended to move into a different class based on their fitness level after the initial class. Andy finds that people always think they are fitter than they are!

Angela Gallagher, owner and personal Trainer at Fitness With Angie in West Des Moines, Iowa, has been teaching and training for over 14 years. Angie trains small groups of women aged 30 to 70. Most have health conditions or chronic joint issues that require careful attention to form as well as occasional modifications. Most are women over 50 wanting to lose minimal amounts of weight, with the primary goal of staying strong, active, and healthy. Angie does a basic fitness assessment

(continued)

In the Trenches *(continued)*

that includes a one-minute crunch test, plank test, and push-up test, and she recently added an elevated burpee test, toe taps, elevated bench jack, elevated push-ups, side plank, renegade rows, and elbow plank. She also measures body fat and BMI and records arm, chest, waist, hips, thigh, and calf measurements. These assessments are included in the price for both personal training and for group classes. Fitness assessments are also offered as a stand-alone purchase.

Summary

Many clubs include fitness and body composition assessments with the membership fees, but one-on-one assessments may be packaged for an extra fee if you own your own studio. Which tests you use may depend on your business structure, the type of setting you're in, and the type of sessions you're offering. To a certain extent, it also depends on your clients—if you train groups that are at a higher risk for SCD, for example, then doing some more in-depth assessments will be a good idea. Ultimately, whether you do any fitness and body composition assessments is your choice. The only "must" is some sort of HRA form such as a PAR-Q+. Remember, different assessments may be necessary for different individuals; assessments should be specific to the needs and goals of each client. Do not retest sooner than four to eight weeks—changes in fitness and body composition take time.

CHAPTER 6

Understanding Your Client and Enhancing the Group Experience

Small-group training is a unique dynamic that can bring out the best in clients through camaraderie and friendly competition. For the trainer, it can also be a lot of fun—or a lot of frustration. Without a good knowledge of motor development and different learning styles, as well as an understanding of the psychology of behavioral change, an SGT session can leave even the best trainers wanting to tear their hair out! This chapter will decrease your frustration by giving you the right tools, including the transtheoretical model of behavioral change (TTM) (Prochaska & DiClemente, 2014), stages of skill development, and multilevel teaching. These will assist your clients in building self-efficacy and help increase motivation and fun.

Having your sessions be a great experience for your clients is one of the keys to a flourishing SGT business. Understanding your clients and their motivations, needs, goals, current level of fitness, and ability helps make this possible. An in-depth knowledge of how skill is built not only makes you a better trainer, but also helps your clients move more efficiently and makes movement safer and more effective. By accommodating all fitness and skill levels, everyone will be successful.

Establish Change Readiness

An essential element of your success will ride on your ability to recognize your client's readiness to change. In the transtheoretical model of behavioral change (TTM), behavioral change is broken down into five distinct stages. The stages can be related to any behavior, but in the exercise context the stages are as follows:

1. *Precontemplation stage.* In this stage, people are sedentary and not even considering an activity program. These people do not see activity as relevant in their lives, or may even discount the importance or practicality of being physically active.

2. *Contemplation stage*. In this stage, people are still sedentary. However, they are starting to consider activity to be important and have begun to identify the implication of being inactive. Nevertheless, they are still not ready to commit to making a change.

3. *Preparation stage*. This stage is marked by some physical activity as individuals mentally and physically prepare to adopt an activity program. Activity during the preparation stage may be a sporadic walk or even a periodic visit to the gym, but it is inconsistent. People in the preparation stage are ready to adopt and live an active lifestyle.

4. *Action stage*. During this stage, people engage in regular physical activity, but have been doing so for less than six months.

5. *Maintenance stage*. This stage is marked by regular physical activity for longer than six months.

Having a working knowledge of the TTM is helpful, but more importantly, it is key to recognize which stage of change your client is currently experiencing. This understanding can guide the types of questions you ask them and how you approach their needs. For example, your client may already be active, but still smokes cigarettes. They may not even be considering quitting; therefore, they are in the precontemplation stage. At this stage of change, providing education about the dangers of smoking and examples of people who've quit can be helpful. Using examples of success as proof that quitting is possible and brings about positive effects may provide the necessary motivation to start thinking about change.

Recognizing which phase your client is in so that you can appropriately coach, motivate, and facilitate behavioral change begins with motivational interviewing (MI), which incorporates empathy and reflective listening to promote honest and open communication. This is especially critical for properly assessing individuals in the crucial precontemplation and contemplation stages, when they are particularly resistant to change.

Here are some questions that utilize MI techniques for clients in the precontemplation and contemplation phases.*

Precontemplation Stage

Goal: Client will begin thinking about change.

What would have to happen for you to know that this is a problem?

What warning signs would let you know that this is a problem?

Have you tried to change in the past?

Contemplation Stage

Goal: Client will examine benefits of and barriers to change.

Why do you want to change at this time?

What were the reasons for not changing sooner?

What would keep you from changing at this time?

What might help you overcome those barriers?

What things (people, programs, and behaviors) have helped in the past?

What would help you at this time?

What do you think you need to learn about changing?

*Questions are reprinted by permission from Dr. Timothy Moore.

One of the biggest mistakes a trainer can make is to assume everyone in their group is at the same state of behavioral change or that change is easy. For many folks, starting and sticking with an exercise program is a complex process. By applying the TTM, trainers can more readily recognize and understand the factors that control behavior and know how to coach new behaviors.

When a client is in the preparation phase, they are ready to take small but important steps toward changing their behavior, including seeking your services. Establishing a schedule, sharing your plan with them, and encouraging them to share their plans on social media or with friends and family can help build excitement and confidence. This builds a relationship of trust that will help move them through the preparation and action phases into maintenance. However, if you skip directly to the action phase without ascertaining the client's specific readiness and needs, you can set them up for failure.

When working with groups, it is important to spend time using MI with each individual during the initial assessment to discover the best approach to designing a targeted action plan. Remember, you can't jump directly from preparation to maintenance without taking clients through the action phase. To move from action to maintenance, it's necessary to create solid support systems while overcoming obstacles or barriers to participation as they arise. Small groups naturally allow for social support; by creating a team environment you can create greater accountability, leading to greater levels of sustained participation. Look for opportunities to celebrate success and treat setbacks or challenges as opportunities for self-improvement. One of the biggest mistakes you can make when moving clients from the action to the maintenance phase is to set up unrealistic goals and expectations. If a client is expecting tangible results in an unrealistic time frame, they are sure to feel like a failure.

Working with clients who are in the maintenance phase in a group with other members still in earlier phases is a challenge that requires great skill and sensitivity. For a client who's established an active and healthy lifestyle, social support through family and friends, smart use of social media, and stress management skills can be extremely helpful. Some of the biggest obstacles to overcome in the maintenance phase involve boredom, distraction, suffering an injury, or overtraining. This is where great program design, multilevel teaching, understanding different learning styles, and working at multiple skill levels can all add up to a greater level of participation for everyone in your group.

Build Self-Efficacy Through the Stages of Skill Development

Self-efficacy is an important motivational element defined as the belief in one's own capabilities—in this case, the capability to successfully engage in physical activity. Self-efficacy influences thought patterns and ultimately how one engages emotionally and behaviorally in all situations. These levels can change very quickly, so when clients feel successful performing each exercise, self-efficacy improves.

Research suggests that people are more likely to be successful in changing their behavior when the change is attempted for positive reasons and associated with positive emotions (Fredrickson, 2009; Seligman, 2002). As a trainer, having the capacity to identify self-efficacy levels in your clients can assist in creating positive experiences. Knowing when to correct movement or when to encourage and motivate can provide clients with exactly what they need to build their self-confidence.

Skill is built through repetition and improves self-efficacy, which ultimately leads to increased participation. This is one of the reasons why skill development is important! In order for a skill to be retained, a movement must be performed often enough for learning to occur. *Skill* refers to movement performed correctly, smoothly, and unconsciously. At any given time different clients may be skilled at different movements. To accommodate these differences, especially when working in a small-group environment, change the exercise only once the skill has been mastered. Create microprogressions for each movement, changing only one element at a time to assure mastery. Changes can be as simple as equipment variations (e.g., switching from dumbbells to rubber resistance cables) or as progressive as adding unstable or dynamic surfaces. Mastering movement progressions builds confidence and self-efficacy! Having your clients finish their session feeling empowered and successful is rewarding. What is critical in order to achieve this success is accommodating the different stages of learning and skill development (see figure 6.1).

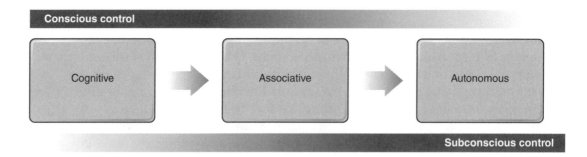

FIGURE 6.1 Stages of skill development.

Cognitive

When a client is initially learning a new movement, they will be at a *cognitive* stage of learning. During the cognitive stage, the client needs to be mentally engaged in order to perform the exercise, and even still, the movement may look jerky and uncoordinated, and the client may make errors.

It's easy to overcoach the client in a cognitive phase, giving them every detail about the exercise. Although counterintuitive, coaching in this phase needs to be kept simple. Too much information is overwhelming and frustrating! The key is to give them just enough information to learn to execute the movement's technique correctly (remember, safety is always the first concern). Over time, skill will be built through repetition. As long as they're performing the exercise safely and properly, with encouragement and good coaching, they will build experience and familiarity. It's important for the client to feel successful to help build their self-efficacy, which can improve confidence and help you retain them as a client.

Associative

The next stage of learning is *associative*. During the associative phase, the client will still be consciously engaged, but to a lesser degree than in the cognitive stage. They are more likely to be more skilled in their movements and have better coordination and timing. They may or may not be fit, depending on whether they are a new learner or a more experienced one returning after a break. They may still need a lower level of intensity even though they move quite well. They are also more likely to have confidence in their movement ability, but not in their ability to stick to an exercise program.

In the associative stage, a base level of skill has already been built, so the client can assimilate a greater degree of information. They might still make mistakes, so communication should be centered on the finer details. Sincere praise for what they are already doing correctly along with the necessary adjustments helps the client in this phase feel successful. Encouragement and enthusiasm can greatly enhance their chances of sticking with it.

Autonomous

Once the skill has been mastered, the client will be in an *autonomous* stage of learning. They are no longer mentally engaged and the movement pattern is automatic. This learner moves smoothly and skillfully, makes few mistakes, and needs little correction. Coaching in this phase involves more motivational strategies than technical instruction. This client can often be partnered with a newer, less skilled client and be given some responsibilities to assist. This can take some of the workload off you and give the more advanced client some motivation.

Within a workout session, a client may be at different levels of learning with similar movement patterns. They may be familiar and skilled at deadlifting but may have never swung a kettlebell. Both exercises utilize a similar functional movement (a hip hinge/bilateral bend and lift), but each involves a different skill set. This means that even though the client may be proficient at kettlebell swings, they may have some new skills to learn to master the deadlift.

Different levels of learning can even be involved with the same exercise. For example, doing a back squat may be autonomous, with smooth movement and efficient technique. Doing a back squat with an Olympic barbell, however, would regress you to a cognitive phase of learning. Even if you're proficient at performing back squats, increasing the load requires much more cognitive engagement.

It's easy to forget what it's like to learn something new, but if you were to try a new sport you would begin at the cognitive stage of learning as well. When working with deconditioned or inexperienced clients, remember that they may need a little more time, understanding, and compassion! Patience and clear vision can help create positive experiences and improve self-efficacy.

Implement Multilevel Teaching

Because small-group training involves coaching two to six people at a time, many of your clients may be at different levels of fitness. This creates a whole set of challenges—not just for your clients, but also for you as the trainer. Coaching groups is an art, not just a practice! Part of this art is being able to recognize the level of learner and provide them with the right level of instruction for the exercise being taught. Making the teaching "invisible" by teaching the base movement first and building from the foundation builds skill and allows everyone to participate successfully.

Novice exercisers often do not want to feel left out and will try to keep up with the other clients in the session. This can create a negative experience for the deconditioned client, who may feel overwhelmed or even injure themselves. By teaching the easiest level first, then offering two or more progressions, the novice learns the appropriate level at which to work and advanced-level exercisers are more likely to perform the exercise with more skill.

Recognizing the learning stage of the client you are working with allows you to effectively communicate the correct level for them to perform the exercise. This may seem very conceptual, but in practice it's actually simple. Figure 6.2 shows an example of a chest exercise, a dumbbell fly. To turn this into a multilevel exercise, begin by keeping the end-level of the exercise in mind, which is the most advanced. For this exercise, the level 3, or advanced variation, has

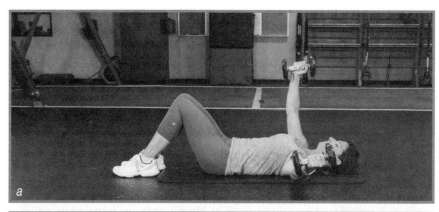

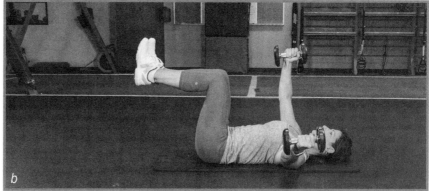

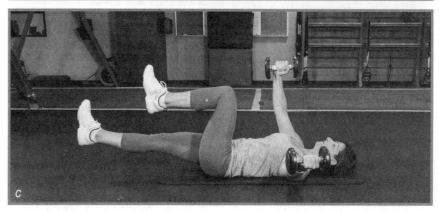

FIGURE 6.2 Dumbbell fly: *(a)* foundational level with feet on the floor and alternating arms (level 1); *(b)* intermediate level with feet off the floor and alternating arms (level 2); *(c)* advanced level with feet off the floor in which the feet alternate with the arms (level 3).

the client lie supine, holding the dumbbells with arms extended (elbows slightly bent) directly above the shoulders, feet off the floor. The movement is performed using an alternating pattern while extending the opposite hip and knee. This asymmetry creates a significant challenge for the core muscles. Breaking it down, the level 1, or foundational level, would be a supine alternating fly with the feet on the floor. The challenge for the core is still present, but the feet on the floor provide stability because of the wider and larger base of support. In the level 2, or intermediate level, the feet are brought off the floor and held there, creating greater instability through a smaller base of support and therefore a greater reliance on the core.

The beauty of the multilevel approach is that each exercise provides the initial strength and basic coordination to build the skill that invisibly "teaches" the next level of the exercise. Keep this in mind when creating your own multilevel exercises to not only assist your clients' strength and skill development, but also to make your teaching easier for a group setting. Starting everyone at the foundational level (level 1) and building from there allows participants to choose which level works for them. Once mastered, the client can self-select to advance to the next variation and so on. Keeping level 1 less complex as well as physically easier is ideal—remember to keep it simple for those in the cognitive stage. Creating greater movement complexity to progress the exercise keeps it interesting and engaging for those moving on to the associative and autonomous stages. The challenge can be increased not just through three different levels of intensity, but also different levels of complexity. Complexity can include changing the base of support, adding dynamic surfaces, creating asymmetry through loading (i.e., using only one dumbbell or cable), or simply by adding more complex movement. Movement can be made more complex by combining upper- and lower-body movements together or adding another plane of motion, such as rotation in the transverse plane (see chapter 9). For example, an unloaded split squat (level 1) could be loaded with a medicine ball and made more dynamic by including a front lunge (level 2), and then rotation can be added as another level of progression. Being able to think on your feet and offer variations will allow each participant to self-select the correct training level. Figure 6.3 provides some guidelines for both progressions and regressions. Most movements can be progressed or regressed according to speed, training surface, load, complexity, and motor and cognitive skills.

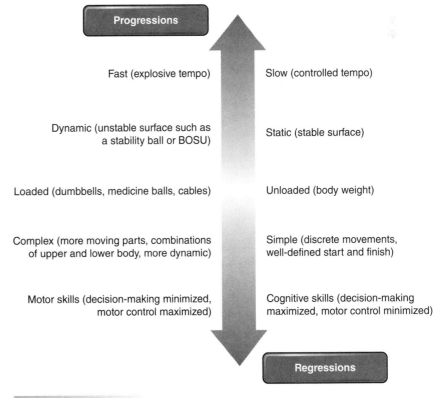

FIGURE 6.3 Guidelines for progressions and regressions.

Data from *ACE Small Group Training Manual.*

USING MUSIC TO MOTIVATE

Playing music in the background offers some free motivation—everyone works a little harder when there's music on! Karageorghis et al. (2011) discovered that music-related interventions bear direct and measurable influence on the brain during the execution of exhaustive motor tasks. Moreover, under the influence of auditory stimuli, affective responses to such exhaustive tasks are altered. This study demonstrated that even high-intensity bouts of physical activity can feel more pleasant under the influence of music, allowing people to train at higher intensities while feeling that it's *easier* to do so.

However, there are some points to be aware of when deciding whether to use music. First of all, music volume, the size and acoustics of your space, and the strength of your voice all play major roles in this decision. Make sure you can be heard over the music! Shouting all day can be exhausting and can damage your voice permanently. Unless you want to exclusively utilize nonverbal communication, keep the volume low enough for you to be heard clearly without shouting. It is critically important that the music volume is kept below 85 decibels (dB) to decrease the risk of hearing damage (a normal conversation in a quiet place is about 60 dB; a chainsaw is 100 dB). If you're in a multiuse facility or a small, shared space, volume and music choices are particular considerations. Keeping the music volume at an appropriate level is important for the courtesy of everyone sharing the space.

Another decision you will need to make is whether you're going to move to the beat of the music. This can, again, be motivating, but will give your class a traditional group fitness feel and can make people who don't like to move to the beat uncomfortable. Using the beat can also create an artificial tempo to the movement you are training. Allowing people to move to their own sense of rhythm and timing creates authentic movement and will encourage your clients to work at their own pace.

The style of music is a final consideration. Make sure the style of music you're choosing is motivating to the clients you're working with—your older clients may not enjoy the latest club mixes. Check to see if people are enjoying it, offer to make a playlist of their favorite songs, and invite suggestions!

In the Trenches

Dr. Timothy J. Moore is a wellness expert who holds a master's degree in exercise physiology and a doctorate in health education. He is a certified strength and conditioning specialist and a Gold Certified personal trainer, as well as one of an elite group in the country who are a Master Certified health education specialist. Dr. Tim has also served as the fitness editor for *Shape* magazine and as a consultant to major companies such as Reebok. His work has been featured in *People* magazine and *USA Today*, as well as on Good Morning America. Dr. Moore states:

The transtheoretical model of change, also known as the stages of change model, is based on solid scientific research, and it provides a sound framework for health and fitness professionals to address the behavior change goals of their clients. Thus you have a comprehensive system that can lead your client on an empowering journey from precontemplation to maintenance in the quest for better health and overall happiness. Just like the American College of Sports Medicine guidelines that personal trainers use to design safe and effective exercise programs, the TTM uses well-established principles to help ensure that the desired outcome is achieved.

Simone Berry is an ACSM-certified personal trainer and a Level 2 TRX coach who trains one-on-one and small groups at Breakthru Fitness in Pasadena, California. Ms. Berry has the following tips for SGT instructors:

Skill level is one of the main things that I consider when training small groups. It's ideal to have participants of a similar skill base, but it's not very common. One of the main ways I handle a group of people with various skills is by partnering people of a similar skill base together. I like partnering people this way because it promotes healthy competition, it gives me time to provide proper instruction to each skill level, and it also makes transitioning through the program more seamless. For example, if one group is performing a barbell squat and step-up superset, partners can switch between the two exercises without having to change the weight on the squat rack. This helps keep them on pace and eliminates unnecessary rest time.

I always employ multilevel teaching techniques because participants are going to be more skilled in one area (e.g., strength) than another (e.g., stability), so even in a one-on-one session I might have to change how I teach an exercise. The way I do this is by having exercise regressions and progressions. The entire group has the same base program and within that program I'll give individual regressions and progressions based on the person's ability.

Summary

Being a great leader goes beyond being a motivating instructor! It also involves being able to understand what stage of change your client is experiencing and where they are in the learning process, as well as successfully coach clients at different levels in the same group. Enhancing the group experience by providing simple, clear, and effective multilevel movement options builds your clients' self-efficacy by allowing each person to progress at their own pace while still feeling included in the group experience. Inclusive, multilevel teaching techniques create cohesion in your groups and help people feel like their needs are being met. This form of communication optimizes the group experience through a deeper understanding of each individual's needs.

CHAPTER 7

The Three Styles of Coaching: Verbal, Visual, Kinesthetic

Clear communication is critical to the enjoyment and success of your small-group clients. An exercise is only as good as how it's performed, so the goal of coaching is to help clients build skill so that movement quality is refined and efficient. However, not all clients learn skills the same way. Not only are there three stages of learning, there are also three primary styles in which people learn: auditory, visual, and kinesthetic.

Auditory learners learn by hearing verbal instructions and often don't need to see the exercise performed. They may say things like "Yeah, I hear you" and "Can you repeat that one more time?" Visual learners learn by seeing demonstrations. They often respond with things like "Oh, I see" or "Can you show me that again?" The kinesthetic learner learns by doing. These learners like to perform the exercise to feel the movement, and with hands-on guidance or a target to aim for, they can self-correct.

Naturally, no one learns exclusively in one style, but people typically have a preference and will learn more easily through one of the pathways. For example, visual learners find having a mirror to watch makes it easier for them to learn, so they can see their form while they move. However, these are the folks who don't always listen! They can seem lost in their own world, making this scenario a frustrating one if learning styles are not taken into account.

The challenge for small-group training comes with the fact that you may have different types of learners at various levels of learning, all performing the same exercises. No easy task! Therefore, a clear demonstration, concise verbal descriptions, and hands-on techniques are ideally used together, with an overlap of all three techniques together to create successful, well-rounded communication. Watch how your participants respond to your instruction. With keen observation you will be able to better understand their learning styles.

Verbal Coaching

Attentional focus examines how mental resources are allocated to create a "flow state" in athletes. The theory states that at any given time an individual's attention can lie at any place along two axes. The first consists of an external or internal focus of attention and the second consists of a broad or narrow focus of attention (Bacon, 1974; Easterbook, 1959; Nideffer, 1992; Watchel, 1967).

Figure 7.1 is an example of how this quadrant may present itself in an SGT class. At any given time, the participant's attention may be external, such as focusing on the instructor giving specific instructions, or internal, such as thinking about how hard the exercise appears to be. Focus may also be broad, such as simply observing other participants doing the exercise, or narrow, such as focusing on what muscles are working in a particular exercise.

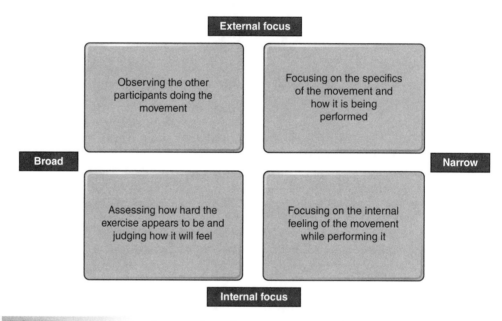

FIGURE 7.1   Internal and external continuum adapted for SGT settings.

Successful verbal coaching for the auditory learner involves creating a framework for external focus. Table 7.1 demonstrates three different external focus cues for four basic movements: a squat, a bent-over row, a push-up, and a plank. Displayed this way, it's easy to see how each cue clearly uses external focus to instruct the basic movement. There are three elements to external focus that you will use to communicate: distance, direction, and description.

- *Distance.* The distance is how far the client should move. Distance can be toward or away, up or down. For example, you might say, "take two steps forward."

- *Direction.* The direction is which way the client should move from an external point of reference (forward, back, right, or left). For example, you might say "lateral shuffle to your left." Direction, for the novice, needs to be cued from a proximal perspective, whereas for the advanced exerciser, distal should be the focus.

TABLE 7.1   External Focus Cues

	Push-up	Bent-over row	Squat	Plank
Cue 1	"Drive the body toward the ceiling"	"Drive your elbow toward the ceiling"	"Push the floor away with your feet"	"Lengthen your spine by pulling your head away from your hips"
Cue 2	"Drive your hands into the floor"	"Crack a walnut between your shoulder blades"	"Squat down as if to sit on a chair just behind you"	"Hold the body rigid like a plank of wood"
Cue 3	"Apply inward pressure between the hands as you press the body upward"	"Stay long as you draw your shoulder blade into your opposite hip pocket"	"Sit back, then as you come up, drive your heels into the floor, pushing downward"	"Pull your navel up away from the floor and toward your spine"

- *Description.* The description uses active verbs, analogies, or comparisons to create the imagery of the intended movement. The description of the exercise needs to be accompanied by a demonstration, including analogies and metaphors to create clarity if necessary: "Hinge forward at the hips, lifting your tailbone, as if to shine your taillights up the back wall" or "Drive your heels into the floor as you press your hips up towards the ceiling, fully opening the front of your hips, like opening a book." See figure 7.2 for a framework for external focus cueing.

There are many different types of verbal coaching beyond the attentional focus framework. By including motivational, positional, alignment, numerical, and mind and body approaches, we can create even more richness to our coaching. Let's take a look.

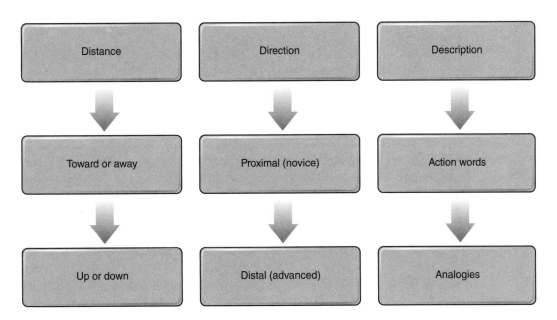

FIGURE 7.2 Framework for external focus cueing.

Motivational

Motivational coaching in a group is definitely different from personal training, and in many respects it's easier. When working as a team, groups do a lot of the motivating themselves. Your job as the trainer is to create the team dynamic by having people work together with your encouragement. Keep in mind that giving people the "why" about the exercise or program can be very motivational. Knowing why you're doing something can ease the discomfort of hard work and make it feel more worthwhile.

Positional

Basic positions for exercises include standing, seated, supine, prone, kneeling, quadruped (on all fours), or side lying. By being consistent in your terminology about position, it can make coaching effective and avoid confusion.

Alignment

Alignment describes where body parts are in relationship to each other (shoulders in relation to hips, knees in relation to feet, etc.). Staying concise and exact when describing correct alignment can cut down on verbal "clutter."

Numerical

Numerical coaching, such as counting reps or using a stopwatch, is potentially powerful—knowing you have only 8 more repetitions or just 10 more seconds can be the difference between pushing through or giving up. But remember, if all you're doing is counting, you're missing a lot of critical information. Many instructors rely solely on endless counting and neglect the motivational or team-building aspects of communication.

Mind and Body

Mind and body communication comes back to attentional focus. Association and dissociation in sport psychology involves focusing attention cues internally or externally during exertion. Association involves focusing on internal cues, such as controlling breathing or maintaining correct form, and can be helpful for improving performance. Dissociation, conversely, involves focusing on external cues, such as listening to music or looking at scenery while running, and has been linked to an improved sense of confidence, relaxation, and enjoyment. Describing when to associate or dissociate ("clear your mind," "focus on your breathing") depends on the context, the goal, and the type of clients you're working with.

To best learn about your strengths and weaknesses, try recording yourself teaching. You may be surprised at what you hear—we are often unaware of our vocal patterns and what bad habits we unconsciously rely on. Remember, rich, effective coaching will include all types of communication. Table 7.2 sums up the different types of verbal coaching and when each is best utilized.

Use this list and make sure your communication covers as many of these elements as possible. For example, when teaching a bird-dog exercise, you could say the following:

> "This exercise, the bird-dog, is great for developing stability in the core muscles while it strengthens the spine to improve posture [motivational]. Come onto all fours, on your hands and knees [positional]. Place your hands directly under your shoulders and your knees under your

TABLE 7.2 Verbal Coaching Categories

Motivational	The "why"
Positional	Where the body is in space (supine, prone, quadruped, standing, kneeling, plank)
Alignment	Where each body part is in relationship to another (shoulders in relationship with hips, knees, ankles)
Numerical	Volume: how many reps or sets; how long to work or recover
Attentional	Coaching the "how" based on an external focus of attention or an internal focus of attention
Mind and body	Association or dissociation; connected or disconnected

hips while holding your head in line with the rest of your spine [alignment]. You will do three sets of four repetitions on each side [numerical]. Start by reaching your opposite hand and foot towards opposite ends of the room [attentional], lifting them up parallel to the floor [directional]. Close your eyes and focus on your breathing; exhale as you lift and inhale as you lower [mind and body]."

Knowing how to recognize an auditory learner is not always simple. Although no one will rely entirely on one of their senses (except in cases of impairment), identifying the predominant learning style is helpful. The auditory learner is the group member who always asks you to repeat yourself or turn down the music so they can hear you. They don't always need a lot of visual reinforcement, so they may not want to stand at the front of the group or in front of a mirror. They are the ones who say, "I hear you loud and clear!"

One of the best ways to improve your verbal teaching skills is to practice giving instructions as if people can't see you. This skill is extremely useful when people are in a position where they are unable to see you without disrupting their exercise, such as at the bottom of a deadlift or bent-over row. Because people often want to watch a mirror, providing them with the right words can help them see the exercise in their mind's eye.

Visual Coaching

In addition to verbal cueing, visual coaching can be added to further relay your message. This time, the key is to teach like they can't hear you—make your gestures big and exaggerated! One of the advantages to visual coaching is that it decreases audio clutter. There is often a lot going on when teaching small groups, especially when you have your group working in partners, if you're outside in a park, or if you have music playing.

Recognizing visual learners when training groups is not as hard as you think. Most people rely on seeing something in order to learn it. These folks are the ones who ask you to demonstrate it again and say, "I see what you mean." They often like to be in the front of the group to get the best view and use mirrors so they can see themselves performing the exercises. They are also the ones who stop moving when you stop and are motivated by you doing the workout with them. For visual learners, having strong body language, great posture, and a powerful presence will help keep them motivated.

Visual coaching can also be particularly helpful with learners in the cognitive stage (see chapter 6). Because this learner is easily overwhelmed, keep the verbal cues succinct and add in some clear nonverbal gestures to decrease information overload. When working with the cognitive learner, simplicity is always the best approach.

When using nonverbal communication, the key is to make your gestures big and emphatic. A simple gesture can be so powerful when used at the right time. Nonverbal communication is most useful when you're reiterating something about an exercise that's both critical and simple. Engaging visual communication techniques should ideally be one simple gesture, like pulling shoulders back while pointing to them; you never want to add a layer that creates confusion or complexity. It could be an alignment cue (like pulling the shoulders back) or something motivational, but no matter what it is, make it big and clear. Table 7.3 provides some suggestions for common gestures you might find helpful.

Keep in mind that it's often critical for the visual learner to see the exercise from all angles. Additionally, it's also helpful to not only demonstrate the whole exercise, but also to break it down into the most important elements. While doing this, be sure to tell them which specific parts they should focus on. A client in the cognitive phase might be so lost or distracted that they don't concentrate when you're demonstrating, so focusing their attention on what is critical can help them learn more effectively. When demonstrating a deadlift, for example, make sure to show it from the side view so clients can see the alignment of the hip, neck, and back. Demonstrate the whole exercise using the chosen equipment, and then again without equipment, specifically bringing their attention to your alignment. Using your hands, point out your hip placement, show neutral lumbar spine, and place a fist under your chin to show neutral cervical spine.

When your clients understand your nonverbal communication, they will do what you want them to do! Naturally, when you start working with a group, backing up your nonverbal coaching with verbal communication can help establish what you're trying to say. If you don't see your clients changing their performance or technique, then it's time to try another form of communication.

Kinesthetic Coaching

The goal of kinesthetic coaching is to have the participant self-correct their faulty movement patterns with methods that make the learning invisible. There are many approaches to kinesthetic coaching, such as hands-on guidance or a target that encourages them to find the path of movement.

When using tactile approaches, make sure you have permission to touch your clients. Always ask first if they are comfortable with it. Make sure your touch is gentle and appropriate and have them move toward a target or your hand—one of the biggest mistakes that a trainer can make is to push a client into position. When you have the client use a target such as your hand or a wall or bench, they not only demonstrate that they are capable of that movement, but they also engage the muscles that are responsible for moving them there. This can make the learning "invisible." For example, when coaching a deadlift, have the client perform the exercise with their back to a wall, lightly touching their glutes to the wall as they hinge forward. This is an excellent way of teaching them to shift their weight back. Next, have them stand several inches away from the wall with no equipment, keeping their feet parallel and knees soft, and perform the deadlift once again. On each attempt, move them

TABLE 7.3   **Common Gestures for the Visual Learner**

Gesture	Utilization
Lifting shoulders up, then pressing them down 	To relax the shoulders away from the ears
Putting hand in front of abs with a fist 	To hold and stabilize the core
Putting hands at the chest and gesturing upward 	To lift the chest
Place your hand under your chin 	To lift the head in line with the spine and align the neck

further away from the wall, until they can only just touch it in the fully lowered position. See figure 7.3 for an example.

Another helpful kinesthetic technique for squats and deadlifts is for the client to hold a dowel rod or light Body Bar touching their back, head, thoracic spine, and sacrum, with one hand holding behind the neck and the other at the lumbar spine. If the head, thoracic spine, or sacrum leave the dowel when the client squats or performs the deadlift, an obvious error has been made. Using this technique during the first session or even just the first set of this exercise can be a simple method of teaching a group. They feel the mistake and are able to self-correct. Again, the learning is invisible! By combining kinesthetic coaching with verbal and nonverbal instruction your clients will have a greater opportunity to learn correct technique. After all, an exercise is only as good as how it's performed. See figure 7.4 for an example.

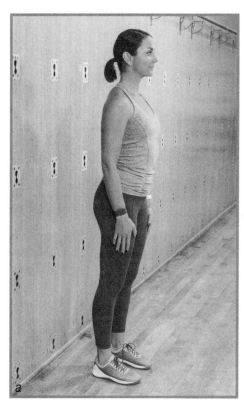
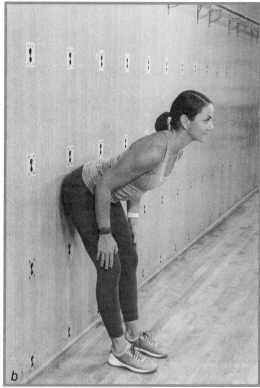

FIGURE 7.3 The client learns by feeling and self-correcting, such as moving their glutes to touch a wall behind them during a deadlift. This example solidifies technique through action.

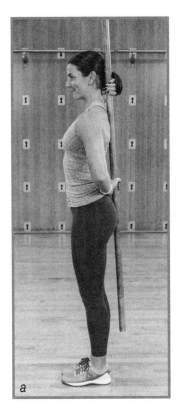
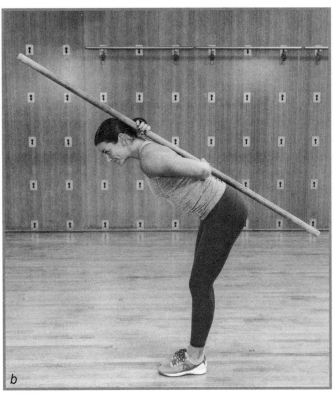

FIGURE 7.4   Place a dowel rod or Body Bar along a client's spine, keeping the head, thoracic spine, and sacrum on the dowel, to automatically place them into a neutral spinal alignment during a deadlift. In this example, they learn by feel.

In the Trenches

Simone Berry, an SGT instructor based in Pasadena, California, has the following advice for accommodating different learning styles in small groups:

> I always pay attention to individual learning styles, which is one of the things that differentiates small-group training from a group fitness class. I show the exercise, give verbal coaching cues, and make form corrections by positioning participants. I try to be as hands-on as possible with my small groups so that they engage with and understand it for themselves. This also comes down to knowing your group. If I know someone learns best by doing something, I try to have them attempt the exercise first and tell me how it feels. That way, when I coach that individual I can use the cues they associate with the exercise.

> One of the things I do to make sure everyone gets attention in the workout is to take notes. This way I know who needs help or adjustments when performing a certain exercise. I don't make a big deal about giving the exact same amount of time to everyone, but I do make sure to connect with everyone throughout the workout. This can be as simple as a touch to correct their form, switching out their weights when they can go heavier, or cracking a joke with someone.

Summary

No matter who your clients are or their level of conditioning or skill, having the tools to teach all types of learners makes all the difference. Keen observation skills, active listening, and engaged coaching can enhance client experience considerably. It takes a keen eye to be able to identify each client's learning style and then communicate effectively for their needs. For effective verbal coaching, simplify your instructions and cue an external focus of attention. This streamlined communication ultimately builds skill, the ultimate goal for any exercise.

Part of creating an amazing and cohesive group experience is to know when to use the different communication styles. Being an effective communicator and motivator for group training goes beyond just instructing and demonstrating; observing and listening also play major roles. By understanding the way people learn, your communication will be more powerful and the teaching will flow naturally!

CHAPTER 8

Strategies to Optimize Group Achievement

K eeping your groups motivated and engaged is important to long-term success. The key lies in your ability to transform your groups from individuals into teams. One of the big advantages to small-group training is that people are no longer accountable to just you; they become accountable to each other. Having people work as a team and support one another creates the kind of synergy that decreases attrition. Building opportunities for teamwork and friendly competition into your workouts can bring out the best in everyone.

In chapter 5 you learned how to minimize risk and assess the level of readiness and fitness for your clients. Once you've gained all pertinent information, grouping your clients based on fitness levels is a great way to promote cohesion and build self-efficacy. However, this is not always possible, so chapters 6 and 7 gave you valuable tools to identify and coach multiple skill levels and learning styles within the group. All of these can optimize group achievement. This chapter will examine further strategies for successful teamwork.

Establishing Rapport

Team building begins with understanding your group and its needs and goals. Once those are established, you need to come up with a plan. Details may involve having enough equipment, making sure the equipment is in perfect working condition, and checking that your space can accommodate everyone and that you can be heard clearly. It's also important that you take into consideration the appropriateness of each exercise for your individual clients—for example, your group members may have similar fitness levels but completely different levels of skill development. Multilevel teaching techniques (discussed in chapter 6) are the key to group success.

Your relationship with your participants is critical. In personal training your ability to build rapport with your clients "is an important determinant of adherence to an exercise program" (Bryant, Green, & Merrill, 2013). Taking the time to lay the foundation of trust and empathy for a new client who may be intimidated can help them build self-efficacy and confidence. Rapport may be the initial deciding factor in whether someone joins your group. Successful trainers consistently demonstrate supreme communication skills, which promotes open communication and the development of trust, which in turn translates into greater levels of participation.

There are three essential attributes needed to develop rapport.

- Empathy
- Warmth
- Genuineness

Empathy is the ability to listen as if you are in the speaker's shoes. It involves experiencing what it's like to be the other person, free of judgments. *Warmth* involves having unconditional positive regard for the other person—not always so easy when some clients might have very different life choices and communication styles than yours. Warmth includes respect and conveys a true level of concern for their needs. *Genuineness* is all about authenticity and having the ability to be open, honest, and straightforward, without putting up a façade. People recognize insincerity. Once you've established rapport it becomes easier to develop a deeper level of trust, an important aspect of the trainer–client relationship. Building relationships with your clients relies heavily on your ability to listen effectively and actively, with empathy and compassion.

Rapport is important in small-group training, but charisma also plays a role. Group training has a different set of demands compared to personal training. The right kind of motivational strategy goes a long way, so understanding your clients' personalities and what motivates them is valuable. Your style of communication will play a role in your retention. There are many types of motivational cues, such as time or rep countdowns, compliments on technique and form, or even emphasizing the emotional or physical benefit of the work performed. These strategies all work well in group settings.

Building a Team Environment

One of the questions you may ask yourself when considering how to build a team environment in your SGT classes is: Why should we be a team? The team environment should make sense and serve the purpose of moving each individual team member toward their goals. Ideally, the purpose of teamwork is to have people reinforce each other through trust and mutual support. Friendly competition in the right environment with the right group can help achieve this. The value of positive reinforcement for sustaining productive results has been established in business settings and sports teams. A great coach is not only an exercise leader, but also a mentor. Tony Dungy, a highly successful football coach and author of *The Mentor Leader*, states, "The mentor leader looks at how he or she can benefit others—which in turn ultimately benefits the individual *and* the organization." Dungy says the "unity of purpose and a desire to make other people better" begins with the attitude and actions of the coach: "It is through that unity or purpose that lives are changed" (2010).

Moving beyond competence to greatness involves having a compelling vision. A vivid picture of where you want to be and what you will look and feel like upon achieving your goals will drive you forward. Staying focused on your vision helps you move beyond setbacks, so you won't quit when the going gets tough. Vision builds perseverance. Create a mission statement to guide you towards your destination, then stay on the path by enjoying the process. To build a team, you need to share your vision, so they too can enjoy the journey.

Having a vision and a mission requires aligning your values to your goals. Your mission statement serves to answer the most important question you can ask: Why do I want to do this? If the answer is aligned with your values—what's important to you as a SGT leader—then this will in turn build your drive. Providing exercise classes is a service that requires putting yourself and your desires aside to best help the people in your groups. In other words, it's not your workout—it's theirs! Instructors frequently make the mistake of thinking that they are getting paid to exercise, but this is not the case. You are being paid to coach, guide, and assist your clients to get the best possible workout, helping them move toward their goals while keeping them safe. A great leader does more than teach; they inspire! An SGT leader must inspire their clients into the state of intrinsic or self-motivation. An inspiring leader is trustworthy, authentic, and competent.

Enhancing the Experience

Great leadership means that constructive feedback and motivation do not come only from you, but from among the entire group. High fives, fist bumps, and cheering each other on to achieve group goals are all opportunities to have the stronger, more experienced regulars in your groups support the newer folks. Inclusiveness is always the goal, so a team-building approach to your sessions will ultimately grow your business. By promoting teamwork, you can encourage your group members to rely on and motivate each other, ultimately fostering adherence. Find ways to create some friendly competition, even against their own previous results. Having a weekly challenge, such as a timed 500-meter rowing race, can be fun and motivating.

Setting people up in pairs or threes for partner and team training also works incredibly well to increase socialization. A fun team icebreaker is to have people share their childhood nickname or favorite sport. Having team members call out encouragement or even naming the teams and creating some friendly competition are further ideas to build friendships and team spirit.

Your ultimate goal is to create an experience that's more than just an exercise class. People seek experiences that make them feel transformed and successful. You don't always know what people are going through in their daily life. The hour they spend with you could be the best hour of their day! Making the class exceptional has the potential to change not only the way they're feeling in the moment, but for a lifetime. Consider the new client who's not sure yet if exercise is enjoyable—your class can begin a lifelong habit of an active lifestyle. Now that's life-changing!

When participants share the experience on social media, it can also help build self-efficacy. Taking photos and posting them on social media provides an opportunity for your team to brag about their achievements. Having your client share their success can make them feel valuable and, in turn, motivate others into action by nudging someone who's on the fence to join your group. It's an important reminder that your responsibilities go beyond developing an effective exercise program. The underpinning of your success lies in creating a memorable, transformational experience.

One of the ways to shape a memorable experience is to encourage participants to celebrate achievements. These celebrations promote a supportive environment and provide further opportunities for team building. Having goal-specific classes and class themes is also a great way to add a fun element. Holiday-themed classes, such as Easter, Christmas, Hanukkah, Halloween, Valentine's Day, or Thanksgiving, can be a winning way to celebrate the occasion and create community. Offering bagels and fruit after a morning class or healthy snacks after lunch or evening classes increases socialization and provides an opportunity for your clients to get to know each other better.

Team challenges with competitive goals, such as Spartan and Tough Mudder races or team triathlons, can also create a sense of working together for something bigger. Designating a team captain, having meetings for planning, creating a team T-shirt, and holding a celebration at the end are all ways of creating community and building bonds with your participants. This all equates to a stronger sense of accountability and helps retain and grow your groups.

Facilitating Goals and Motivation

Participation in your SGT classes is driven by the client's experience, so staying centered on their goals helps them not only achieve success, but also assists them in enjoying the process. Meaningful goals ideally provide the framework for that process. Specific, measurable, attainable, relevant, time-based goals, or SMART goals, create that framework.

Specific Goals

Specific goals need to be quantifiable. Vague statements such as "I want to get in better shape" don't create enough focus. Instead, have clients write down their specific goals, such as "I want to get fit so I can run a 10K," or "I want to lose 15 pounds." A specific goal can also involve improving sleep, decreasing stress levels, or lowering cholesterol and blood pressure. Help people narrow their goals to two or three main objectives, then break down the small steps that move toward achievement. For instance, if a 15-pound (6.8 kg) weight loss is the goal, then breaking it into small increments of 1.5 pounds (1 kg) per week will be less daunting and feel more doable.

Measurable Goals

Goals should be measurable, so that you can track their progress. Measurement can be either subjective or objective. It could be pounds lost, back pain decreased, or even self-esteem improved. Subjective measurable goals are typically centered on feelings, whereas objective goals are more externally measurable, such as being able to run a 5K race.

Attainable Goals

Attainable goals must be realistic! These goals take into account the individual's training experience, current level of conditioning, and intensity of their motivation. People frequently have unrealistic ideas of how quickly goals can be attained because magazines and celebrities are constantly selling instant weight-loss supplements or programs that guarantee miracles. Instead, you should help your client set attainable goals through education and clear explanation.

Additionally, a client may decide on a specific and measurable weight-loss goal by committing to an exact number of sessions per week, and then they get a new job that doesn't allow time for as many sessions as they originally planned. Programs need to have enough structure to promote adherence, but if they are too rigid, they may elicit guilt and feelings of failure. Therefore, to help the individual be successful, goals need to be attainable.

Relevant Goals

For a client to make significant changes in their lifestyle, like getting more active and joining your SGT classes or committing to modifying their diet, goals have to be relevant to them personally. This is where goal setting needs to be collaborative; it's not good for you to set the goals if they are not meaningful to your client! To make a commitment to change, the goal must have personal relevance.

Time-Based Goals

Time-based goals should have a deadline. This helps motivate clients to get started and stay focused. Set a long-term goal, then create some short-term stepping-stones to help them be successful. Short-term goals assist clients in seeing progress along the way.

ESTABLISHING GROUP GOALS

Setting overall team goals can help create cohesiveness within your groups by lifting up the lower performers and helping the higher performers achieve a sense of accountability. For example, if you're utilizing rowers for circuit training, you could set a group goal based on meters rowed by the entire group for the time period. Set a specific amount of time, such as two minutes, and have each of the team members row at a maximum intensity for that interval. Record the distance for each person and then add all the distances up to tally the winning team. The same idea can also be performed on a bike with a power meter. Set a distance goal of a quarter mile per person, add each member's time, and see which team finished the fastest. With the right group of participants, these competitions can be a great system for team building and bonding.

Identifying Motivational Strategies

Identifying motivational strategies for your clients is an important aspect of good coaching. There are two basic forms of motivation: intrinsic and extrinsic. Intrinsic motivation is internal—being driven by feelings such as a desire for accomplishment or enjoyment of the process. Extrinsic motivational strategies are external and may include rewards, incentives, and recognition. If you're working with a group of new exercisers, having a leaderboard of accomplishments is one way of providing some recognition and thereby extrinsic motivation.

Although extrinsic motivation compels short-term compliance, intrinsic motivation is more favorable for long-term adherence to a new activity. For this reason, it's a good idea to transition beyond extrinsic rewards to intrinsic motivation after the initial six months of training. The art lies in knowing where your group is in their fitness journey and then providing the appropriate motivation strategies. Keep in mind, these strategies can be used before, during, and after your SGT sessions. Look for opportunities to support your new participants with things like text message reminders before the sessions and acknowledge them for their efforts during the sessions. Branded T-shirts, hats, and workout towels can be offered as incentives for signing up for a specified number of sessions or achieving specific milestones. These small incentives can provide some extrinsic motivation to new folks.

For your more experienced regular participants, try to emphasize inner motivation such as workout satisfaction, feelings of success, or simply how good it feels once the workout is done. For both the new and experienced exerciser, making the change feel smaller by breaking it into smaller chunks of work can motivate your groups. John Wooden, a former UCLA basketball coach, once said: "When you improve a little each day, eventually big things occur. . . . Don't look for the quick, big improvement. Seek the small improvement one day at a time. That's the only way it happens—and when it happens, it lasts."

To facilitate intrinsic motivation, allow your clients to develop skill mastery with each exercise before progressing to more difficult variations in complexity and intensity. As your group masters movement progressions, they will achieve a sense of accomplishment. To assist in this process, it's important to emphasize that expectations should be realistic. Help your groups recall previous successes and remember their feelings of satisfaction. Continue to emphasize the benefits of being consistent with class participation to help build adherence. By emphasizing accomplishments, you can build self-efficacy. Having clients watch each other perform an exercise can provide additional intrinsic motivation: "If they can do it, so can I!"

Preparing for Your SGT Sessions

For a new instructor, coaching a small group of individuals can feel intimidating. Being fully prepared, organized, punctual, and focused will help guide your success. Being prepared means having a solid workout plan. Here are some questions to ask about the class:

- Can the exercises be taught at multiple levels?
- Is the class plan suitable for the group goal and appropriate to meet individual needs?
- What is the fitness and skill level of most of the group?
- Do I have enough equipment for everyone?
- Is that equipment in perfect working order?
- Is my space free of clutter?

Being punctual is also critical. If you're early, you're on time. If you're on time, you're late—and if you're regularly late, you have little chance of success! Starting and finishing the class on time is not optional; it's a matter of respect for your clients' time and part of being organized and professional.

Finally, focus makes you a much more effective coach. Your ability to guide and motivate groups also lies in being motivated yourself. Make sure you're getting adequate sleep and taking care of your fitness and wellness needs. Are you eating a balanced diet and staying hydrated? Are you taking time off from work and finding balance in your lifestyle? These are all important considerations. An effective coach is 100 percent present, which requires staying healthy and focused.

In the Trenches

Brett Klika, CSCS, IDEA Personal Trainer of the Year, and cofounder of SPIDERfit Kids (spiderfit-kids.com), is well known for his ability to create camaraderie and is an expert in team building. He offers the following tips for building group camaraderie:

> In any group situation, it's important that the leader proactively creates a positive group dynamic. This begins with simple things like making sure everyone in the group knows each other and is able to call each other by name. Additionally, through the course of a training program, the leader should facilitate games, activities, and even events outside of training that increase interaction. As a leader, one needs to be sensitive to individuals with bold personalities that attempt to dominate the group. This can interfere with creating effective camaraderie.

> My number one tip for team building is to present activities that highlight different strengths. When a member of a team feels they have something to contribute, and the other members recognize this unique contribution, it bonds a team. When training, consider presenting games and other challenges that provide opportunities for all participants to be successful. For example, in any group, there is usually one individual who is the most skilled or fit. Presenting an activity that incorporates trivia, problem solving, spelling, geography, or math provides opportunity for someone else to be highlighted. This also demonstrates different strengths among participants. This becomes part of a group identity and is highly effective for creating camaraderie.

> In the fitness industry, one of the biggest challenges for instructors is client retention. Once we get clients, keeping them feeling valued, accountable, challenged, and engaged is just as much of an art as a science. A group situation is ideal for improving accountability. In order for the small group to be successful, however, all members must feel comfortable, valued, and competent. Facilitating a team dynamic that allows for camaraderie will improve adherence, and ultimately, client retention.

Summary

Encouraging team dynamics, establishing group and individual goals, and building intrinsic motivation and self-efficacy will ultimately optimize how your group works together. Cohesion is the key to motivation and consistency. Creating the type of teamwork that builds and models healthy competition provides support for your newer members and promotes leadership in your established participants. By seeking every opportunity to foster that teamwork, you will deliver a memorable experience that goes beyond leaving sweat on the floor.

PART III

APPLYING FOUNDATIONAL TRAINING PRINCIPLES TO PROGRAMMING PRACTICES

CHAPTER 9

Programming Components and Training Variables

One of the most exciting elements of training is the body's ability to adapt to virtually any stimulus. It's these very adaptations that help clients get the sort of results they seek. Understanding programming principles and knowing how to manipulate the training variables makes this change possible. However, knowledge is not the same as having practical application skills; this is where the sample programs and sidebars in this book come into play. This chapter will help you bring your workouts to life using the teaching and communication skills you learned in chapters 6 and 7.

Here you're provided with the foundational information you'll need to help your clients get results, along with ideas for how to construct effective programs for your classes. When the principles are correctly applied, working out is no longer a random series of exercises put together without true purpose, but instead a logical progression that leads from foundational skills to a more advanced training stimulus. The exercise and program progressions will help you develop appropriate programs for your classes based on sound principles.

Specificity, Overload, and Progression

A resistance training program is planned around the needs, goals, and current condition of the clients. Effective, long-term adaptation to a resistance training stimulus is guided by key principles that allow the body to adapt to the stress response from resistance training. This stress response can be created by a manipulation of the three primary principles of resistance training. These three principles are *specificity, overload,* and *progression.* The goal of exercise program design is to manipulate the variables of specificity, overload, and progression for a desired outcome. This creates a training overload and causes physical adaptation.

Principle of Specificity

Our body adapts to the specific demands imposed on it. This principle of specificity is critical to understand! The specific adaptation to imposed demands (SAID) principle of training means that, for example, when a client works with barbells, their body will adapt to that stimulus, then when the same exercises are performed with dumbbells, they will readapt. Each change of equipment is a different stimulus and each new exercise provides a different training overload, even when using the same muscle group.

This also means that when transitioning new clients from machine-based training into a small group with different equipment, there will be a whole new set of adaptation challenges. Balance, coordination, body control, and stabilization are new constraints that the individual needs to develop in order to perform skills correctly. For a client who's been training on a machine, the pads of the machine stabilize and hold the body in place, the arms of the machine guide the limbs, and although strength is built, less control, stabilization, or balance is involved. Transitioning the client to standing exercises with elastic resistance bands means that loads need to be lighter, communication needs to be clear and concise, and exercise progressions and regressions become critical.

The beauty of the specificity principle is that when training with simple exercises that represent functional movements found in daily life, such as squats, lunges, pushing, pulling, and rotational movements, an improvement in elements like coordination, balance, and body control is seen, thereby enhancing sports performance or activities of daily life. Clients who train functionally will naturally develop more coordination, body control, and balance, leading to greater movement efficiency.

Principle of Overload

To produce desired adaptations to a training program, the variables of the exercise program must be manipulated to create an overload on the physiological systems of the body. Overload can be achieved by increasing the load, increasing the volume (number of reps or sets), or decreasing rest between exercises or sets. In other words, for training to be effective, it's necessary to drive the body to work harder than what it's used to doing. The level of overload must be appropriate to the training experience and fitness level of the clients. When this principle is not correctly applied, injuries are more likely to occur. Muscles gain strength more rapidly than tendons and ligaments, so appropriate loading is an important consideration. For deconditioned and inexperienced clients, less intensity can provide adequate overload.

Volume is defined as the total amount of work performed (weight lifted) during an exercise session. It is generally expressed as a product of intensity × sets × number of repetitions. The total volume of a workout must be dictated by training experience and goals of the clients. Volume increases time under tension (TUT), which provides the training stimulus for muscular hypertrophy. Greater volume also requires greater amounts of time and should therefore be considered when planning your classes. Most critical is the fact that high-volume training is a natural progression and is unsuitable for novice exercisers. When training deconditioned individuals, lower workout volumes are more appropriate.

Intensity is defined as the specific amount of resistance or external load applied to muscles. If the same resistive force is consistently applied, then the muscle will not be stimulated and a training overload will not be created. Intensity is written as a percentage of the maximum amount of weight lifted for one repetition, or one-repetition max (1RM). Greater intensities increase motor unit recruitment and muscle force production, which translates into gains in *strength* and *power*. The external load must also be appropriately applied. Again, for deconditioned individuals, less intensity is more appropriate. For those groups, lower percentages of the 1RM are important to prevent injuries. As clients gain experience, greater levels of intensity can be tolerated and are necessary to continue making gains. Experienced clients will benefit from training at higher percentages of the 1RM.

Table 9.1 is an example of the training outcomes for different volumes and intensities. This table is based on a periodization model of training, which means that a client begins with muscular endurance before moving to the next phase of training. Each training phase could take anything from three to eight weeks before progressing to the next phase. Remember that progressions in intensity and volume should always be in small increments. Even with strength as the goal, starting a novice exerciser at greater than 85 percent 1RM would be inadvisable. A good place to start would be to set a goal of improving muscular endurance, then building to the development of larger muscle mass, before moving to true strength training. The foundation must be built before progressing to greater increases in intensity and volume to ensure that ligaments and tendons are also ready for increases in intensity. Each phase has specific, goal-oriented variables of intensity and volume. Although this table may look confusing at first glance, a progressive training scheme is one of the keys to preventing overtraining or injury.

TABLE 9.1 Training Outcome Recommendations for Repetitions, Sets, and Intensity

Training goal	Repetitions (per set)	Sets (per exercise)	Intensity (%1RM)
Muscular endurance	≥12	2-3	<67%
Hypertrophy	6-12	3-6	67%-85%
Strength	<6	2-6	>85%

Adapted by permission from NSCA, "Program Design for Resistance Training," by J.M. Sheppard and N.T. Triplett, in *Essentials of Strength Training and Conditioning*, 4th ed, edited by G.G. Haff and N. T. Triplett (Champaign, IL: Human Kinetics, 2016), 458, 463.

Principle of Progression

A training overload must be achieved in order to trigger changes. To create the safe and effective overload necessary to facilitate adaptation, the intensity, volume, and movement complexity must be increased gradually over time. Allow adequate time for adaptation before progressing to more challenging levels of intensity, volume, or movement complexity. If this principle is not adhered to, there is a high likelihood of injury.

Progression must always be appropriate to the goal and fitness level of the client. Movement complexity and skill level of the clients is also an important component of progression to bear in mind. Progressions with small, incremental changes allow time for adaptation, so as not to physically and psychologically overwhelm your groups. Change only one element at a time and only alter the exercise once the client has mastered it. Remember that dramatic increases in intensity can be counterproductive, even to the advanced-level exerciser.

Periodization

Resistance training programs consist of numerous variables, including load (intensity), volume (reps and sets), frequency, rest interval, exercise selection, and exercise order (Williams et al., 2017). Periodization is defined as planned, cyclical (i.e., the program repeats) manipulation of these resistance training variables to attain peak performance at specific times of the year (Evans, 2019). In small-group training, an important consideration may be that load is not always a variable that can easily be manipulated. Bodyweight exercises and commonly used equipment such as rubber resistance bands and suspension training systems limit how much load can be added; therefore other variables (volume, rest interval, exercise selection, and exercise order) may need to be adjusted for SGT programming when considering the objectives of the group.

Periodization training originated in sports with an annual competitive season, which require different levels of training volume, intensity, and specificity; these variables are manipulated depending on the competition schedule and the athlete's goal. The method was developed to prevent overtraining, help prevent plateaus, and build optimal performance and fitness for the competitive season. Evans (2019) cites research indicating that lengthy periods of training that lack variation results in stagnation and fatigue. Consequently, one of the main purposes of periodization is to provide structure to the variability in the training components to decrease the likelihood of a plateau or decline in physical (and mental) performance. The success of periodization in sports has brought the protocol into mainstream fitness settings and with smart planning, can be incorporated into SGT settings.

There are three basic periodization models: linear, block, and undulating or nonlinear. The two focused on here are linear and undulating. The training cycles are broken into phases that focus on one or more goals. The phase length can vary from sport to sport, depending on the length of the general physical conditioning, sports-specific training, and competitive season. For general conditioning for small-group training, the phases for linear periodization may be as follows:

- Microcycle: Single training session or one week of training
- Mesocycle: Two to three weeks of training
- Macrocycle: Four weeks of training

In SGT settings, a macrocycle may be four to eight weeks, depending on how you set up your training schedule, the goals of the group, and the type of people you work with. It may also follow linear or undulating formats, depending on your clients' needs and goals. Each of the microcycle goals move toward a common mesocycle goal, and the mesocycle goals aim for the overall macrocycle goal. This type of training plan works well for closed sessions, in which you have continuity and consistency with your groups. Figure 9.1 provides an example of a four-week macrocycle, within which there are two two-week mesocycles and four one-week microcycles.

Figure 9.1   Four-week macrocycle periodization model

Macrocycle 1 (4 weeks)	Mesocycle 1 (2 weeks)	Week 1: Microcycle 1
		Week 2: Microcycle 2
	Mesocycle 2 (2 weeks)	Week 3: Microcycle 3
		Week 4: Microcycle 4

Linear Periodization

The phases of training for linear periodization change load (intensity), volume, frequency, and rest in sequence according to the goals of each phase. This strategy starts with high volume, low intensity and then progresses to low volume, high intensity (Grgic et al., 2017). Each phase builds toward the next, thereby creating a foundation for the increases in intensity and volume in the subsequent stage. Theoretically, the initial high-volume phase provides the stimulus for hypertrophy and the later high-intensity period challenges the neural mechanisms in the body (Kok, Hamer, & Bishop, 2009). This cyclical manipulation of the training variables allows the body to adequately adapt to each phase. See figure 9.2 for a sample of how the phases are broken down using linear periodization.

Figure 9.2   Typical linear periodization progression model

Macrocycle (4+ weeks)	Mesocycle (2-3 weeks)	Microcycle (1 week)
	Mesocycle 1: Muscular endurance	Build general muscular endurance, with low force and higher volume (2-3 sets of 12-15 reps)
	Mesocycle 2: Muscular hypertrophy	Muscular hypertrophy involving higher volume and varying loads (3-5 sets of 6-12 reps)
	Mesocycle 3: Muscular strength	Muscular strength, with highest load and lower volume (3-5 sets of 3-6 reps)
	Mesocycle 4: Muscular power	Explosive training, with high load, lower volume (3-5 sets of 2-4 reps)

Undulating Periodization

Undulating periodization involves frequent alterations in volume and intensity within a training program; these alterations often occur weekly or daily (Evans, 2019). When employing undulating periodization, each microcycle focuses on one specific goal: This could be high intensity, low volume, or low intensity high volume, for example. Evans's research indicates that undulating periodization programs are likely the best choice for strength development. McNamara and Stearne (2010) propose that undulating programs have the advantage of a decrease in overtraining and mental boredom while allowing the greatest adaptability to travel or possible disruptions in the training program. Linear periodization doesn't allow flexibility in this way. The training variables can be applied in any order according to your clients' needs and goals, offering greater flexibility in their application.

The advantages of undulating, or nonlinear, periodization in small-group training are many, especially for drop-in open sessions that don't lend themselves to ongoing participation. It allows greater flexibility for the participants because it's not as strict as a linear model. Undulating periodization has been studied in moderately resistance-trained women. Pelzer, Ullrich, and Pfeiffer (2017) researched the training effects of an undulating periodized program with 19 female college-aged students (none of whom were competitive athletes), and determined that both linear and undulating periodization programs were effective at producing hypertrophy in a time period of four to six weeks. In a unique study, De Souza et al. (2018) examined different patterns in muscular strength and hypertrophy adaptations in untrained individuals undergoing nonperiodized and periodized strength regimens. It was determined that in the latter part of a training program (after the initial six weeks) the periodized regimens elicited greater rates of muscular adaptations compared to non-periodized regimens, and that periodized regimens might be advantageous at latter stages of training even for untrained individuals.

Figure 9.3 is an example of a four-week macrocycle utilizing an undulating model with a focus on hypertrophy. As illustrated, there are more hypertrophy workouts than strength or endurance. The emphasis can be changed based on the group goals. If your group has a six-week macrocycle, two more microcycle weeks would be added.

Figure 9.3   Four-week undulating macrocycle periodization model emphasizing hypertrophy

Macrocycle (4 weeks)	Mesocycle 1	Microcycle (week 1)	Monday: Endurance Wednesday: Hypertrophy Friday: Strength
		Microcycle (week 2)	Monday: Hypertrophy Wednesday: Strength Friday: Hypertrophy
	Mesocycle 2	Microcycle (week 3)	Monday: Endurance Wednesday: Strength Friday: Hypertrophy
		Microcycle (week 4)	Monday: Hypertrophy Wednesday: Strength Friday: Hypertrophy

Endurance: General muscular endurance, low load and higher volume (2-3 sets of 12-15 reps)
Hypertrophy: High volume and varying loads (3-5 sets of 6-12 reps)
Muscular strength: Highest load and lower volume (3-5 sets of 3-6 reps)

Ultimately, whether you decide to employ some sort of periodized plan in your training is based on the type of business model you have set up (closed or open session), your clients' goals and needs, and the type of equipment available (heavier loads versus body weight). Studies that favor the results gained from a periodized model; clients' goals, your business model, and available equipment may dictate whether or not periodization is appropriate. The programs outlined in this book offer a good starting place to manipulate the training variables and provide a periodized model of training that fits your clients. Use the basic structure of each plan, then vary the volume, intensity, exercise order, exercise selection, and rest interval to suit the needs and goals of your clients.

Movement-Based Training

Movement-based training, also known as functional training, is useful for individuals of all ages and abilities. It's important to understand how all the body's systems interact and work together, whether it's finding a balance between the relationships of joint stability or appreciating how the body can create compensations for weakness. Recognizing how each system can support the enhancement of fitness and decrease the potential for injury assists trainers in designing goal-specific programs.

Elements of Human Movement

When broken into its raw components, human movement is a blend of multiple elements, with each intrinsically linked to the next—stability and mobility; coordination and balance; strength, flexibility, and endurance; and a motor program (see figure 9.4). This cyclical linkage means that each element is dependent on the other. If any of these elements are missing, movement efficiency decreases. Movement-based training builds whole-body coordination, which in turn enhances the stability and mobility relationships, which improve strength, flexibility, and endurance, which in turn will develop balance and the motor program. Ultimately, this entire cycle boosts fitness and well-being and decreases the potential for injury and movement deficiencies.

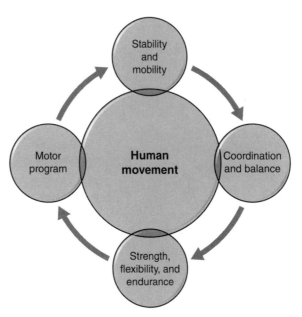

FIGURE 9.4   Elements of human movement.

Stability

Stuart McGill, a spine research expert in sports and fitness and author of *Low Back Disorders*, states that stability is "your ability to maintain your posture and balance while moving your extremities" and that "increasing stiffness of the muscles increases stability and increases ability to support larger loads without failing" (2002). Training for stability is synonymous with core training. One mistake frequently made by trainers when core training is using static exercises, in which the position is sustained, the extremities are stationary, and the exercise is made more challenging by increasing the duration. However, as McGill succinctly put it, "while moving your extremities" is the key to training the core. Instead of simply holding the position, increase the intensity by moving the arms and legs through different planes of motion.

Mobility

Mobility allows the body to move fluidly, promotes good posture, and provides flexibility. Mobility is flexibility in action and can best be described as the synergistic actions of the skeletal joints and neuromuscular systems to allow uninhibited range of movement around a joint. Mobility is also dependent on joint structure to provide this freedom of movement, however, it must never compromise joint stability. For example, a ball-and-socket joint has greater mobility than a hinge joint. Just like stability, mobility allows the body to move efficiently. For professionals who sit for a living, whether behind a computer or the wheel of a car, the high volume of low-amplitude movement creates huge imbalances between stability and mobility. These are the folks who most need mobility training!

Balance

In order to have efficient human movement, balance is critical, particularly for the active older adult. Including exercises that challenge your client's ability to maintain their center of gravity over their base of support, both dynamically and statically, is essential for preventing falls. Beyond mechanical balance, training the body to have good symmetry between opposing muscle groups can assist in injury prevention.

The human body's segments have a natural tendency to be either more stable or more mobile based on how they need to function. For example, the foot needs elements of mobility but also needs to be stable enough to push off during the gait cycle. The ankle needs to have excellent mobility in all three planes of motion, whereas the knee is a hinge joint, a naturally stable structure, moving primarily in the sagittal plane. The lumbar spine is also a stable structure, with the facet joints designed to only have one degree of freedom, providing only limited movement in the sagittal plane. Further up the spine is the thoracic spine, a mobile structure that has three degrees of freedom and movement in all three planes to allow full mobility for activities of daily living and many sports. The problem many clients have is a lack of mobility in their mobile structures, leading to overcompensation in the stable structures. For example, if a client has a thoracic spine that's locked down and immobile due to a desk job, chances are they will not only have an upper back problem, but also a lower back and shoulder problem. This is due to the law of facilitation.

Figure 9.5 demonstrates the rhythm and balance between the body segments and joints from the foot to the shoulder. All the joints exhibit

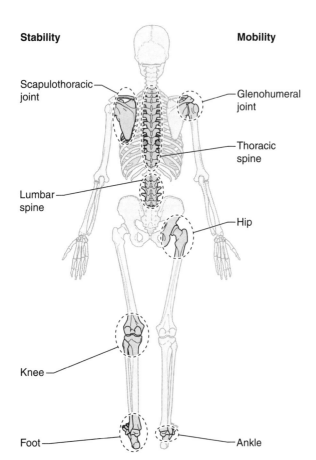

Stability | **Mobility**

Scapulothoracic joint
Glenohumeral joint
Thoracic spine
Lumbar spine
Hip
Knee
Foot
Ankle

FIGURE 9.5 Stability–mobility relationships.

THE LAW OF FACILITATION

When examining the human movement system, there is one additional element to consider: the law of facilitation. This principle is based on the idea that the human body will facilitate movement along the path of least resistance and will move habitually through the same path of motion, even when there is a lack of movement efficiency. These compensatory movement patterns become so ingrained that the individual may not be conscious of the habit. Think of someone walking with a limp. Without being aware, they favor one side of the body and their gait changes to accommodate pain and the movement pattern then becomes habitual.

It's also important to consider how this affects the stability–mobility relationships of the body. When a mobile joint lacks mobility, the body will facilitate that movement from the stable structure above or below in another plane of motion. This further disrupts the motor program, and smooth, coordinated, efficient motor patterns develop into movement compensations. For example, a knee problem is frequently caused by an ankle's lack of mobility, forcing the knee to move into other planes of motion. It's easy to look at the symptom and not the cause, but by understanding the relationships between stability and mobility, you can begin to unlock the secrets behind the causes of many of the body's compensatory tendencies.

Considering these relationships is important for exercise selection, program design, and injury prevention. Although the individual goals of group training make this more challenging, all human bodies function similarly. If you run a corporate wellness program, for example, you may have weight loss, stress reduction, and strength gain as individual goals for each client, but most of them sit for a living and will therefore have related stability and mobility issues.

different levels of stability and mobility based on joint structure and function. Ball-and-socket joints are naturally more mobile, whereas hinge joints are stable. The facet joints of the lumbar spine are primarily stable and have only small amounts of movement, which occur mostly in the sagittal plane.

Strength

The ability to apply maximal force against gravity or resistance can be considered a good general definition of strength. Strength is an important element of fitness that should be developed in order to prevent age-related sarcopenia, or the loss of muscle mass after the age of 35. As the human body ages, sarcopenia can also cause a general overall decrease in mobility. Most research agrees that sarcopenia involves the loss of type II (fast-twitch) muscle fibers first, which means movements are not as powerful or quick. This in turn can increase the likelihood of a fall, because the body has to react quickly and powerfully to a loss of equilibrium. Therefore, maintaining or gaining muscular strength is an important goal for most fitness and wellness programs.

Flexibility

Optimal flexibility allows the body to move through a functional range of motion. In other words, you could say that people need to be as flexible as they need to be for what they do. A gymnast, for example, needs extreme levels of flexibility for their sport, yet a runner needs much less flexibility. If you were to compare the flexibility demand differences between a marathoner and a sprinter, however, you'd see that a sprinter also moves through much larger ranges of motion compared to someone who runs distance. When designing flexibility into your programs, you must consider what function that range of motion will provide for your clients' activities of daily living and potential sports performance.

Endurance

Endurance is the ability to maintain or continue muscular contraction or cardiovascular movement. In cardiovascular terms, the heart, lungs, and vascular system are being trained to improve efficiency. With so many benefits to enhanced cardiovascular conditioning, it's an essential element of health, fitness, and well-being. Muscular endurance training targets type I (slow-twitch) muscle fibers, which function for most sustained activities (e.g., postural stability). Many isometric core exercises train these muscles to sustain a desired specific position, such as prone or side planks. Even if traditional strength or hypertrophy are the program goals, maintaining muscular endurance for different areas of the body is valuable.

Motor Program

Motor program, or coordination, is the ability to move efficiently and as intended. When the body is trained as an integrated whole, the motor program is also trained as a direct result of these unified movement patterns. As skill is developed, there is a greater capacity for work because the client is able to train with greater efficiency.

Patterns of Human Movement

Human movement can be broken down into five primary patterns:

1. Bilateral bend and lift (i.e., squat, deadlift, hip hinge)

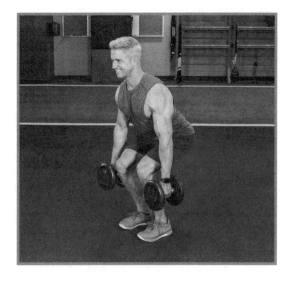

2. Single-leg stance (i.e., gait, lunge, step-up, single-leg squat)

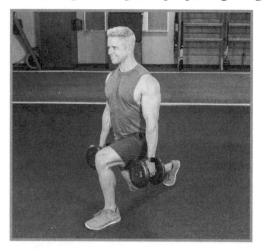

3. Horizontal or vertical push (i.e., shoulder and chest musculature)

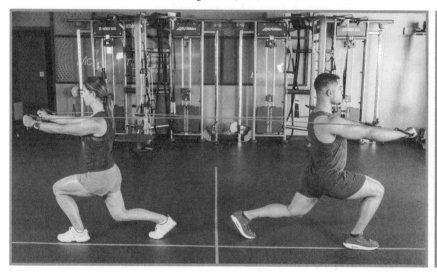
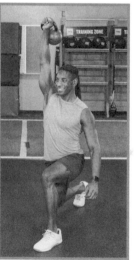

4. Horizontal or vertical pull (i.e., shoulder and back musculature)

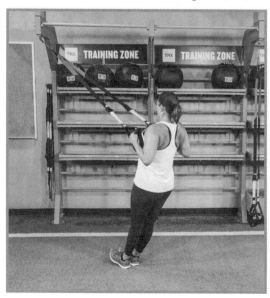
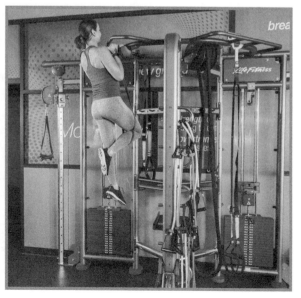

5. Rotational and spiral movements (i.e., rib cage and pelvis moving in sync or out of sync)

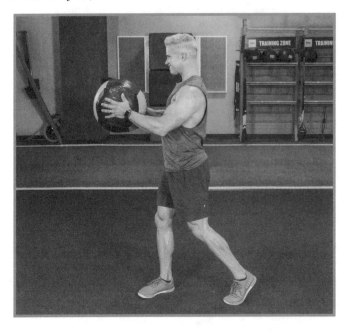

When movement-based training is the primary focus, each of these movement patterns should be included to enhance coordinated strength. A balanced and complete program will include all five patterns through all planes of motion. By balancing the planes of motion with all five movement patterns, improved muscle symmetry is the outcome.

Three Planes of Human Movement

As an SGT instructor, it's critical to understand the application of the planes of motion. Because different muscle groups work in different planes of motion, it's important to create a program that trains the body through all planes to effectively train muscular balance. Training in all planes adapts the body more effectively to all activities of daily living and sports performance. The three planes of human movement are frontal, sagittal, and transverse (see figure 9.6).

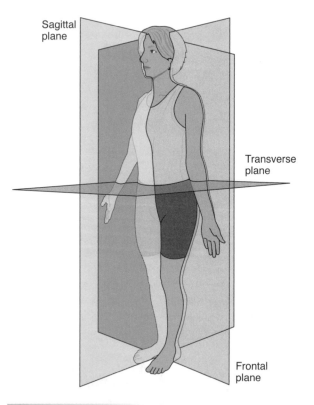

FIGURE 9.6 Planes of human movement: frontal, sagittal, and transverse.

MOVEMENT TRAINING: TRAINING FOR ENHANCED FUNCTIONAL ABILITY

Movement-based exercise has become a mainstream method of training and has many benefits beyond simple aesthetics. The goal of this type of training is to improve the way the body moves in daily life and sports performance. The transference from the gym to activities of daily living (ADL) is the key and overall goal. Open kinetic chain exercises train specific muscles often in supported environments with machines that stabilize the body, such as a hamstring curl or knee extension. Even with machine-based training there are significant cocontractions of the stabilizing muscles, so while the goal of many of these exercises is to train a single muscle group, there is more than an isolated training effect. Closed kinetic chain exercises, or weight-bearing movements, are typically more integrated, with the goal of more than a single muscle group being overloaded. These movements incorporate ground reactive forces and gravity and typically involve dumbbells, cables, medicine balls, and the like. Coming back to the example of a squat, the gluteal, quadriceps, hamstrings, adductors, abductors, core, and lower leg muscles are all functioning together, with eccentric, concentric, and isometric cocontractions at different times during different phases of the movement.

Therefore, when deciding between machine-based workouts and free-standing movement-based training, examining the goal and outcome is an important factor. When focusing on an integrated exercise program, think in terms of what movement pattern is being performed rather than what muscles are being trained. The irony lies in the fact that while the focus is on the pattern of coordinated movement, muscles are trained. It's a different perspective. Multimuscle, multiplanar, multi-joint movement is the path to providing enhanced movement quality, coordination, and total-body control. Train these movements, and the muscles will adapt.

Consider the body as an orchestra, with the muscles as instruments and the nervous system as a conductor. If each musician practices alone, the sound would be anything but harmonious. But when the orchestra practices together, following the conductor, the music is harmonious. When training for movement, the nervous system is always conducting the quality and contribution of each muscle or muscle group. The nervous system is always involved for balance, proprioception (the ability to sense where your limbs are positioned in space), stability, and coordination—all critical elements in movement efficiency.

For the sagittal plane of motion, imagine yourself standing in an extremely narrow hallway with your shoulders trapped between the two walls. Walk straight down the hallway and you will be moving in the sagittal plane, using hip and shoulder flexion and extension. Next, imagine you're standing sideways in that hallway, with the walls pressed to your front and back. Move only between those walls using abduction and adduction, and you'll be moving in the frontal plane. Finally, if you picture a hula hoop moving around your waist in circles, you would need to move your hips in a circle to hold it up. This rotational movement of the hips is an example of a transverse plane motion.

Table 9.2 shows joint actions and exercise examples to further clarify the planes of motion.

TABLE 9.2   Planes of Motion, Joint Actions, and Movement Examples

Plane	Joint action	Example
Sagittal	Flexion	Concentric biceps curl
	Extension	Eccentric biceps curl
	Plantarflexion	Concentric calf raise
	Dorsiflexion	Eccentric calf lowering
Frontal	Abduction	Concentric lateral raise
	Adduction	Eccentric lateral raise
	Elevation	Shrugging shoulders up
	Depression	Pressing shoulders down
	Upward rotation	Scapular rotating up
	Downward rotation	Scapular rotating down
Transverse	Rotation	Russian twist or wood chop
	Internal rotation	Transverse lunge stepping in
	External rotation	Transverse lunge stepping out
	Pronation	Hand or foot rotating down
	Supination	Hand or foot rotating up
	Horizontal flexion	Concentric cable fly
	Horizontal extension	Eccentric cable fly

Plyometrics

Plyometric exercise falls into the power phase of training, which is the most advanced phase and has a high caloric expenditure. Plyometric exercises rely on the myotatic stretch reflex within the muscle spindle. The myotatic stretch reflex responds at the rate a muscle is stretched, which causes an equally rapid contraction. Muscles briefly store the tension developed by rapid stretching so that they possess a potential elastic energy. Plyometric exercises enable a muscle to reach maximum strength in as short a time as possible. The amortization phase, the moment of time between the lengthening and shortening phases, is extremely fast.

When incorporating plyometric training techniques, it is essential to consider your clients' level of fitness. Plyometrics are naturally complex and intense, involving explosive, high-impact exercises. This means that they need to be applied during the more advanced phases of training, such as during the power phases.

Plyometrics are not recommended for clients who have osteoporosis or are deconditioned. Although they offer a high caloric expenditure and a high level

TRAINING FOR FUNCTION: PROGRAMMING CONSIDERATIONS

When designing a training program with the goal of improving movement ability, exercises should focus on the five primary movement patterns. Typically, the equipment will include tools such as dumbbells, cables, medicine balls, resistance bands, or even body weight. The whole purpose of such a program is to help the body adapt to movements that have a high transfer into activities of daily living, such as a squat, deadlift, or step-up, which would enhance the ability to get out of a chair, pick up something heavy off the floor, or walk up a flight of stairs. Integrated training is ideal for almost anyone. The exception would be inactive, older, frail, or deconditioned adults, especially those with balance deficits or osteoporosis, for whom a fall could incur a high risk of injury. Consider the following when planning a movement-based approach to training:

1. Focus on integrated movement, rather than isolated, single-joint exercises, such as a squat or lunge.

2. Introduce multijoint movement that occurs in multiple planes. Machine-based training typically allows only a single plane of motion, such as a seated knee extension versus a multidirectional lunge.

3. Build complexity in a progressive manner. Integrated movements are typically more complex because they involve multiple movements through multiple planes. This may make it necessary to break the movements down into smaller components for learners in the cognitive stage of learning (see chapter 6 for more on stages of learning).

4. Build intensity in a progressive manner. Integrated training involves more muscles working together, so it can be more intense. This intensity may need to be built gradually, either within the workout or over time.

5. Focus on the functional ability to stabilize and generate force from the core. This is a huge advantage over isolated, single-joint training because functional movements will train the body to recruit the core throughout the workout in ways the core is naturally utilized.

6. Develop movement patterns that have high transfer to natural activity. This builds a body with a purpose: a body that can move efficiently and achieve desired goals.

7. Balance the planes of motion. Different muscles work through different planes of motion and they must be balanced to create muscle symmetry. This in turn builds a body with good proportion and decreases overuse of specific muscles.

8. Incorporate all planes of motion. Many people come to the gym and think they're doing the right thing by training opposing muscle groups and while this will always be important, it may end up being uniplanar. They might do a leg press, a knee extension and hamstring curl, a chest press, a seated row, a biceps curl and triceps extension, a back extension and trunk curl—and they trained with every movement in the sagittal plane! Now imagine if that person played tennis on the weekend: Because tennis is a multiplanar, multidimensional weight-bearing sport, that person is likely to be injured in the planes of motion they didn't train.

of intensity, consider whether these types of movements are appropriate for your clients before incorporating them into your classes.

Plyometric Exercise Definitions

A plyometric exercise can be broken down into five categories of movement. All of these explosive movements utilize the stretch–shortening cycle of a muscle contraction (the muscle spindle). For example, before a jump, it's necessary to squat down (eccentrically load) before taking off (concentrically unload). It's almost impossible to jump up explosively without first squatting, making the movement fall into the category of a plyometric exercise. The plyometric categories are as follows:

- *Jump*: Take off from both feet and land on both feet simultaneously
- *Bound*: Take off on one foot and land on the opposite foot
- *Hop*: Take off from one foot and land on same foot
- *Throw*: Concentric acceleration of an object with an upper extremity, or an explosive push
- *Catch*: Eccentric deceleration of an object with an upper extremity, or a rapid deceleration

Plyometric Intensity Classifications

Plyometric exercises can be classified into three major categories: low intensity, moderate intensity, and high intensity. These classifications are based on the level of impact as well as the complexity of the movement; therefore, movements with higher impact are considered higher intensity. Plyometric movements should be introduced to participants who have higher fitness and skill levels. The safety of these types of movements rely on the client's ability to eccentrically decelerate, or land from a jump correctly and efficiently. For example, if a client squats with a valgus knee alignment (knees bending in toward the center line of the body, or knock-kneed), then a squat jump would be a poor choice of exercise. The following is a description of the categories:

- *Low intensity*: Single linear jumps or jumps in place, such as jump rope exercises or a boxer's shuffle (small bouncing movements from foot to foot)
- *Moderate intensity*: Multidirectional jumps or multiple linear jumps, such as drills on an agility ladder or mini-hurdles
- *High intensity*: Depth jumps or hops and bounds, such as box jumps or high-hurdle jumps or hops

Movement Efficiency

As previously mentioned, it is nearly impossible to perform an explosive movement, such as a jump, bound, or hop, without first eccentrically loading the muscle, usually by bending and lowering the body. This reflex is what makes explosive movement powerful and efficient; it utilizes the elastic properties of a muscle contraction. Figure 9.7 provides an outline of the stretch–shortening cycle of a muscle contraction.

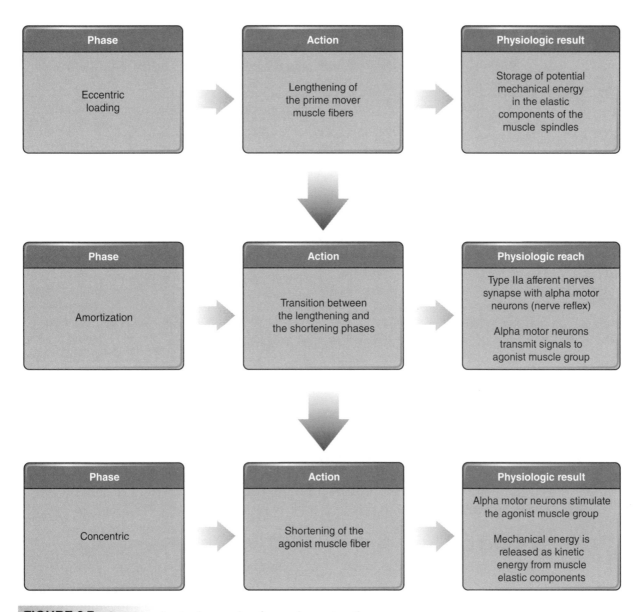

FIGURE 9.7   Stretch–shortening cycle of muscle contraction.

Variables of Exercise Program Design

Your exercise program can be designed through the manipulation of the variables and based on the goals, fitness, and skill level of the participant. Variables include specificity, volume (sets, reps, and load), and intensity (1RM), all of which can influence the overload and progression. One of the main differences between traditional group exercise and small-group training is the goal specificity of the workouts. The workout variables of small-group training create the overload specific to the needs and goals of the participants, thereby creating a program tailored to the clients. Traditional group exercise classes often have more generic goals to allow for the wide range of participant needs. It is this specificity of training in small groups that adds value for participants. Table 9.3 defines the variables of exercise program design.

TABLE 9.3 Variables of Exercise Program Design

Variable	Definition
Intensity	The percentage of 1RM (one-repetition max)
Repetitions	The consecutive number of times an exercise movement is performed before resting
Sets	The total number of repetitions performed before resting
Volume	The total amount of work performed during an exercise session (intensity × sets × reps)
Tempo	The speed of the repetition (velocity of movement), which determines the time under tension (TUT) of muscles involved (the slower the movement, the higher the TUT)
Rest interval	The rest period necessary between sets (the heavier the load, the longer the time needed for rest; the lighter the load, the shorter the time needed for rest)
Training frequency (recovery)	The number of training sessions within a specific time frame; adequate recovery is necessary for adaptation to occur and to allow the muscles to recover from fatigue
Exercise selection	The exercise movements chosen to allow for proper motor learning, skill acquisition, and exercise adaptation

There are also several other variables to discuss here. By using these variables, it is easy to progress or regress the training intensity, complexity, and overall difficulty, especially when equipment choices and load availability are limited. Some of these provide training stimuli that can enhance core stability, balance, mobility, and other secondary fitness attributes.

Leverage

Leverage can be defined as the application of force through rigid objects (levers). The human body is a system of levers (bones) and fulcrums (joints) that allows us to manipulate objects in order to achieve movement goals, such as lifting a box off the floor. There are three basic classes of levers: first, second, and third.

Much of the human body operates with third-class levers, in which the muscle force acts between the resistance and the fulcrum. Figure 9.8 shows an example of a third-class lever, such as a biceps curl.

A second-class lever, designed to lift very heavy forces, places the resistance between the muscular force and the fulcrum. Figure 9.9 shows a second-class lever, such as a calf raise or a wheelbarrow. In the example of a heel raise, the ball of the foot is the fulcrum, the resistance is the body weight, and the force is the attachment of the Achilles tendon.

A first-class lever is one in which the fulcrum is positioned between the muscle force and resistive force, such as a seesaw (see figure 9.10). This type of lever is not typically found in the human muscular and joint system.

Changing the lever length of an exercise can change the intensity of the exercise without changing the load. For example, a push-up performed on the knees has a shorter lever than a push-up performed on the toes. In this

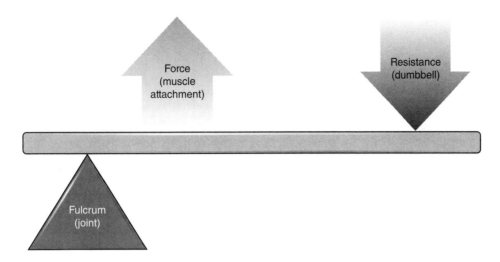

FIGURE 9.8   Third-class lever (biceps curl).

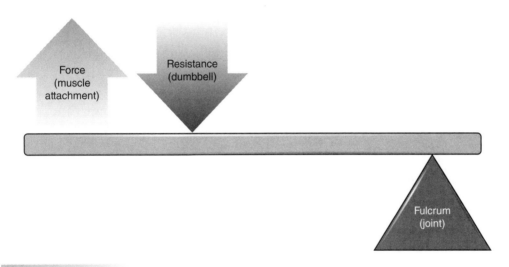

FIGURE 9.9   Second-class lever (calf raise or a wheelbarrow).

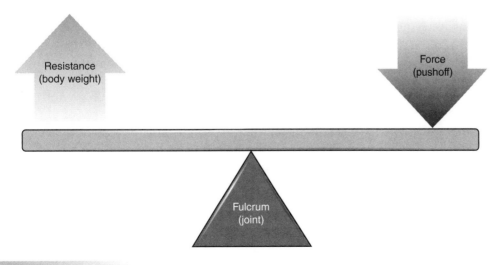

FIGURE 9.10   First-class lever.

example, the shoulder joint is the force, the feet (or knees) are the fulcrum, and the body is the lever. This makes the movement a second-class lever. The further away you hold load from the fulcrum (the joint closest to the center of the body), the greater the force around that joint.

As another example, holding a 10-pound dumbbell with the arm fully extended, level with the shoulder, feels extremely different from holding that same amount of weight with the arm hanging down by the side. By extending the arms and holding the hand further away from the body, the lever length increases; therefore, the intensity or loading on the joint also increases. This variable is especially effective when training with small devices such as medicine balls, kettlebells, dumbbells, and rubber resistance bands. When training groups with small, portable devices, manipulating the lever length is a great option to increase intensity when adding an external load is not an option.

Asymmetry in Loading

In traditional training it is common to load both sides of the body symmetrically, especially when using machines. However, consider loading only one side—the imbalance produces forces through the core in order to compensate, which is an effective way to further stimulate trunk musculature.

Partner Training

Having a partner is a fun and social way to train. Creating an environment of teamwork can definitely help build your business by enhancing interpersonal relationships between your clients. From a practical standpoint, it can also mean you need less equipment. Partner training is also an advantage when using rubber resistance bands, because they allow the user to establish an external anchor point, providing diverse lines of pull (one of the main drawbacks of rubber resistance bands is that the equipment must be anchored on the individual's body, such as around a foot, which not only prevents the user from moving their feet, but greatly limits the exercise selection and effectiveness).

Equipment Variations or Combinations

With so many great equipment choices available, trainers have a ton of options. Varying the equipment for your groups can create a whole new level of stimulus and thereby create a training overload to provide results. Small, portable equipment is inexpensive and typically offers more functional exercise options. Consider too that your clients can supply their own equipment. For example, if you'd like to use stability balls, you could stipulate that each client supply their own. This not only solves the financial burden for you, but also the storage or transport issue of having four to six balls. It also allows you to set "homework" for your clients because they have equipment! No matter how you set up your business and what the group goals are, the right equipment can help your clients succeed.

One way of setting up your business is to have an equipment-specific group, such as a kettlebell training group or a TRX boot camp. This type of training plan can attract a very specific population looking for that type of workout and can set you apart from other businesses.

Use of Momentum

Momentum, the tendency of an object in motion to continue in motion as outlined in Isaac Newton's first law of inertia, can be utilized specifically when it comes to training the body. Many basic human movements and sport movements rely on momentum (i.e., running, or swinging a baseball bat). Momentum allows us to move forcefully and efficiently. While traditional strength training is typically performed with slower, more controlled movements, some exercise techniques, such as a kettlebell swing, rely on a dynamic motion, and, therefore, momentum. When momentum is harnessed intentionally without the loss of body control and with smooth coordinated movements during exercises such as a correctly-performed kettlebell swing, then momentum is valuable. The value comes from being able to control the momentum, and this takes a combination of stability, mobility, strength, and flexibility.

The problem arises when working with deconditioned groups who lack body control and coordination. This is when momentum ends up not being harnessed intentionally! Therefore, it may be more appropriate to train with control and avoid using momentum with individuals who lack body control. However, using momentum strategically with the right people can be extremely effective: Adding explosive movements can increase intensity, caloric expenditure, and complexity as well as provide a progressive element to a workout. When used appropriately, this advanced technique can take a workout to the next level. This is especially useful for clients involved in sports that require momentum. By training with environmental similarity, there is greater carryover to enhance movement efficiency and performance.

Exercise Order

Changing the order of the exercises can enhance motivation and prevent boredom while still allowing your group to build skill by keeping movements consistent. This provides your group the opportunity to improve motor skills while adding a new stimulus to the workout. It can also feel like a whole new workout even though it's the same equipment and exercises! By adjusting the order of movement complexity or the exercises themselves, the training stimulus is changed, providing a fresh overload.

The max power exercises and multijoint movements should be performed at the beginning of the workout and single-joint isolations at the end (if you're using that mode of training). Include exercises that involve multiple muscles toward the beginning of the workout, when your clients have the greatest amount of energy. This can help them get the most benefit from these types of movements and decrease the risk of injury due to neural, synergistic muscle, or stabilizer fatigue. For instance, if you train your biceps to fatigue before doing a set of chin-ups, your client will struggle with the chin-ups since the bicep muscles are a synergist (assistant muscle group). If the goal is to fatigue the latissimus muscles with a multijoint movement like a chin-up, then the biceps will be too fatigued to assist. Similarly, if you train the core muscles to fatigue before performing back squats (with a barbell on the back of the shoulders), the fatigued core muscles may not be "available" to stabilize the back and an injury may occur.

Base of Support

Changing the base of support can dramatically alter the level of difficulty of an exercise. By taking the same exercise and gradually decreasing the base of support, you can create a practical progression while enhancing balance, core stability, and kinesthetic awareness. There are four basic stances on a continuum from most stable to least:

1. Staggered stance, with feet wide in a split stance, provides stability in both the sagittal and frontal planes.
2. Square stance, with feet parallel and shoulder-distance apart, provides stability in the frontal plane but less so in the sagittal plane.
3. In-line stance, with one foot directly behind the other as if on a balance beam, provides stability in the sagittal plane but very little in the frontal plane.
4. Single-leg stance, the most advanced position, offers multidirectional instability.

Unstable Surfaces and Devices

Stability balls, BOSU balls, and other dynamic surfaces add an immediate progression to basic exercises. They also add an element of fun and play. This equipment provides a huge training stimulus to the proprioceptive system for balance, stability, and motor control. Keep in mind that balance can also be effectively trained on stable surfaces with changes in base of support. Base-of-support changes can also be used to progress and regress work on dynamic surfaces by adding an additional contact point, such as holding a dowel or wall. Almost all populations can train with these devices with some variations.

Even newer to the fitness world are water-filled devices and other dynamically loaded equipment offering top-down instability. Rather than standing on an unstable device and manipulating a stable object, instead stand on a stable surface and manipulate an unstable object! The idea of a dynamic, shifting load is to stimulate proprioception, balance, and core strength, as well as excite the nervous system and promote transference into daily activities and sports performance.

In the Trenches

According to Paul M. Juris, Ed.D. Human Movement Scientist and Health & Wellness Pioneer, when approaching program design from a functional perspective, it's important to remember that "function" is related to the outcomes of the program and not necessarily the processes. Fundamentally, does the program produce the desired results, regardless of the methods that were employed?

This is relevant, especially in today's empirical scientific environment, in which evidence-based practices define our methodology. But here's the challenge; when we look across the broad spectrum of science that addresses functional outcomes, we're confronted with a wide array of disparate methods, each of which is effective in producing results. In simple terms, there's more than one way of achieving an outcome.

So, how do we determine the most appropriate methods for small groups, or individuals, participating in a program of functional development? The answer is not by choosing the best formula or recipe, but by improving our mastery of the foundational sciences that underscore human movement. By learning the tenets of human movement science, we empower ourselves to better identify real issues, make critical decisions and create solutions that result in measurable improvements.

Summary

When you understand the why, the how is much easier! Having foundational knowledge provides insight into how to effectively train small groups. Small groups have a different set of requirements compared to personal training or traditional group exercise. This makes understanding the science even more important. It may not be possible to create a truly personalized program design, but with a sharp eye and clear knowledge, compromises can be minimized. The application of the training variables must always be appropriate to the needs, goals, and current condition of your group, but just remember that the principles of science will always apply and you will have the potential to be effective and successful with all of your clients.

CHAPTER 10

Advanced Training Techniques

Advanced training techniques such as high-intensity interval training (HIIT), metabolic training (MT) and lactate threshold training (LTT) are becoming increasingly popular in the mainstream fitness market. Multiple scientific studies are available to back up the methodologies of these techniques and guide professionals in how to maximize their benefits, which include rapid increases in $\dot{V}O_2$ and positive changes in body composition.

Small-group settings offer a perfect opportunity to utilize these techniques, especially for those groups who have already established above-average levels of fitness. Studies on deconditioned individuals have also shown positive results, although it may not be advisable—these clients are likely to find these techniques too demanding. For groups with superior levels of fitness, however, it can offer the perfect progression and an additional challenge. Always keep in mind that training must be appropriate for and suitable to the needs and goals of your groups, but with careful application within a periodized scheme, advanced training techniques can be truly beneficial.

Advanced Training Modalities

Once your clients have achieved a reasonable level of fitness and are seeking additional challenges, you may consider introducing advanced training modalities. For individuals with high self-efficacy seeking to further their fitness, continuing to train at the same degree of intensity may leave them feeling bored and unengaged. As the saying goes: "If you want something you've never had, you've got to do something you've never done!" Furthermore, for clients who have already reached their goals, utilizing advanced training modalities can help them maintain their gains. The three main approaches discussed here are high-intensity interval training, metabolic training, and lactate threshold training. Later in the chapter, we will also cover some additional ideas for other advanced techniques you're sure to find applicable.

High-Intensity Interval Training

High-intensity interval training (HIIT) uses high-intensity cardiovascular intervals alternated with active recovery intervals. The workouts typically include short bursts (6 seconds to 4 minutes) of intense exercise (≥90% maximal aerobic capacity) alternating with relief breaks of varying lengths (Boutcher, 2011; Kessler, Sisson, & Short, 2012).

Various HIIT protocols and their metabolic outcomes are outlined in table 10.1. These protocols vary among intervals of various lengths with recovery bouts that are less than, equal to, or greater than the work effort. As you can see, many studies have demonstrated that HIIT induces numerous positive physiological adaptations that resemble traditional endurance training, despite a low total training volume. Because lack of time is most frequently cited as the reason for not exercising, this is exciting news.

The application of these techniques in small-group training may involve plyometric bursts or the utilization of HIIT on machines. With many of the studies performed on a cycle ergometer, it would be simple and effective to add an exercise bike as a station to circuit training formats. Treadmills and rowing machines are also a great addition to circuit training, especially because rowing is a total-body exercise that quickly adds intensity and increases caloric expenditure. The studies noted in this chapter demonstrate that these high-intensity intervals have a huge impact on fitness levels and metabolism making them an effective addition to advanced training programs. However, there are a few important biological factors to consider.

When exercising at low intensities, levels of blood lactate remain relatively stable. When maximally employing the glycolytic system, blood lactate levels rise markedly. The lactate threshold (LT), or anaerobic threshold, is reached when the body cannot remove the lactate at the same rate it's being released. Although $\dot{V}O_2$max sets the upper limit of aerobic energy production, it is the LT, or an individual's metabolic level, that determines the percentage of $\dot{V}O_2$max used within a certain amount of time (Coggan et al., 2010).

TABLE 10.1 Influential Studies of HIIT Training

Study	Warm-up	Interval timing	Intensity	Volume
Tabata, Nishimura, Kouzaki, Hirai, Ogita, Miyachi, et al., 1998	15-20 min; bike protocol	20 s:10 s	170% of $\dot{V}O_2$max; Recovery incomplete	8 sets = 4 min of work
Gibala et al., 2012	10-15 min; bike protocol	30 s:~4 min	All-out cycling effort against a supramaximal workload	4-6 work bouts for a total of 2-3 min of intense exercise during a 20-min session
Iaia, Rampinini, & Bangsbo, 2009	8-15 min; running protocol	10:20:30 x 5 reps; 2 min between sets	90%-95% of $\dot{V}O_2$max 50%-60% of $\dot{V}O_2$max 25%-30% of $\dot{V}O_2$max	5 sets = 25 min of work
Tremblay, Simoneau, & Bouchard, 1994	8-15 min; submaximal bike protocol	15 s:60 s or 30 s:90 s	60%-70% of $\dot{V}O_2$max; Recover HR to 120-130 BPM	10-15 sets = ~8 min 4-5 sets = ~12 min
Perry, Heigenhauser, Bonen, & Spriet, 2008	8-15 min; bike protocol	4 min:2 min	90% $\dot{V}O_2$max	10 sets = 60 min

The body also relies on two energy systems: the aerobic and the anaerobic energy pathways. Because the body will always find a way to transfer (produce) energy, when the demand for adenosine triphosphate (ATP) is higher than what the aerobic system can produce, the body shifts into anaerobic metabolism. HIIT training is specifically designed to tax the anaerobic system. Table 10.2 provides an example of different activities and the energy demands involved.

TABLE 10.2 **Energy System Continuum**

ATP-PC system	ATP-PC and LA system	LA and O_2 system	O_2 system
Anaerobic		**Aerobic**	
Shot put Javelin High jump Long jump 100-meter sprint Base stealing Golf swings Tennis swings	200- and 400-meter sprints Football (halfbacks, full-backs) Speed skating 100-yd swim Velodrome cycling	800-meter dash Gymnastic events Boxing (3 min rounds) Wrestling (2 min periods)	Soccer Lacrosse Cross-country skiing Marathon Jogging Many cycling events

Adapted from E. Fox and D. Mathews, *Interval Training: Conditioning for Sports and General Fitness*, (Sanders, 1974).

ACUTE PHYSIOLOGICAL RESPONSES TO A HIIT WORKOUT

HIIT training produces some immediate and significant physiological responses that have a huge impact on fitness, body composition, and the endocrine system. HIIT elevates the sympathetic nervous system while depressing the parasympathetic nervous system. With growth hormone increasing up to 10 times above baseline, it is easy to see why HIIT training is so effective at decreasing body fat levels while increasing lean muscle mass. The following list describes the effects of a HIIT workout on the body (Boutcher, 2011). It's important to note that the degree of these outcomes depends on the volume and intensity of the training session.

- Heart rate elevates significantly
- Epinephrine and norepinephrine are elevated 6.3 to 14.5 times above baseline
- Blood glucose from glycogen breakdown is initially elevated for exercise fuel, but may decline during the HIIT session
- ATP and phosphocreatine decline steadily (used to meet rapid fuel needs of contracting muscles)
- The sympathetic nervous system, which speeds up neural messages, is elevated
- The parasympathetic nervous system, which slows neural signaling messages, is depressed
- Lactate levels may increase up to 10 times above baseline
- Growth hormone may increase up to 10 times above baseline
- Venous blood returned to the heart is enhanced, directly increasing stroke volume
- Increased levels of blood glycerol and free fatty acids suggest early breakdown of triglycerides

Metabolic Training

Metabolic training (MT) is an advanced training format that consists of compound, whole-body exercises with little to no rest between sets in order to maximize caloric expenditure in as short a time as possible. Metabolic training focuses on increasing metabolic rate during and after exercise. A typical MT workout may incorporate alternating upper- and lower-body repeated supersets, known as *reciprocal training,* before moving to the next superset. For example, a workout may consist of four different supersets, each performed for three to four sets. The first superset may be a squat and chin-up, followed by a lateral lunge and a push-up. This may be followed by a step-up and a push press, and the fourth superset might include a single-legged deadlift and a cable row. Here are some guidelines:

- MT uses large muscle groups through a large range of motion (ROM)
- MT is high intensity, typically training to momentary muscular failure
- MT increases metabolism postexercise through increased excess post-oxygen consumption (EPOC)

Lactate Threshold Training

It's important to understand the value of training at different intensities. Lactate threshold training (LTT) is unique compared to HIIT and MT. Remember, when exercising at relatively low intensities, levels of blood lactate (a metabolic byproduct produced during the breakdown of carbohydrates) remain reasonably stable (Robergs, Ghiasvand, & Parker, 2004). When maximally employing the glycolytic system, blood lactate levels rise markedly. The lactate threshold (LT) is the fastest a person can continuously run, cycle, swim, or aerobically exercise in a steady state bout without fatiguing (for up to an hour, depending on the fitness level of the individual). In essence, it is a person's maximal steady state of continuous exercise. LT has been identified in research as the best predictor of endurance performance (McGehee, Tanner, & Hourmar, 2005). If it is exceeded, fatigue will ensue much sooner (McGehee et al., 2005). The real culprit of acidosis, or "the burn," is the accumulation of H+ ions in the muscle contractile environment. It is now known that lactate actually buffers the acidity in the cells by accepting H+ ions within its biochemical structure that would otherwise impair exercise performance.

Lactate threshold training is essentially training the body's physiology to be more resilient in its production of lactate. It is therefore valuable for clients to train at or close to LT to improve lactate buffering; if the pace at LT can be increased through training, then race times will invariably decrease. In other words, an athlete can run faster without working harder which is a huge advantage for clients who are training for and competing in endurance events such as 5K races, sprint-distance triathlons, or even mud running obstacle courses. All of these types of short-duration high-intensity endurance events require high levels of fitness and a high LT. Furthermore, training at LT has been shown to induce advantageous physiological adaptations that increase endurance (Dalleck & Kravitz, 2003).

Table 10.3 provides a sample LTT workout that can be performed on any type of endurance training equipment, such as a stationary bike, rower, or treadmill. This type of workout is intended to attain and sustain a threshold intensity for a given period of time. The goal is to sustain the threshold using heart rate (HR), ratings of perceived exertion (RPE), and watts (if your machine measures wattage). For HR, the threshold intensity will be at around 80 to 85 percent of maximum HR (HRM); RPE will feel hard to very hard.

Because it's extremely uncomfortable to sustain an effort at threshold intensity, coaching and motivation is critical. Having some music in the background can help with the motivation and atmosphere. Remember to be precise with your timing; this way you can build trust with your group. As always, watch each participant carefully for any signs of overexertion or overheating. Hydration reminders are also a good idea.

An RPE guide for this LTT workout is as follows:

- *Easy (55%-65% HRM)*: Conversational pace, can easily maintain a conversation, breathing is through the nose and mouth and very comfortable
- *Moderate (65%-75% HRM)*: Can speak a sentence but not a paragraph, breathing through the nose and mouth, no longer comfortable to breath only through the nose
- *Hard (75%-85% HRM)*: Can only speak a few words, breathing is uncomfortable, and the pace can be sustained (threshold)
- *Very hard (85%+ HRM)*: Breathless, unable to speak, and the pace cannot be sustained

TABLE 10.3 Sample 45-Minute Lactate Threshold Training Workout

Modality	Intensity	Time
Warm-up (12 min)	Easy	2 min
	Build to moderate	4 min
	Hard/moderate intervals	30:30 s × 4
	Easy	2 min
Interval 1	Hard	Sustained 4 min
Recovery	Easy	2 min
Interval 2	Hard	Sustained 4 min
Recovery	Easy	2 min
Interval 3	Hard	Sustained 4 min
Recovery	Easy	2 min
Interval 4	Hard	Sustained 4 min
Recovery	Easy (allow full recovery to rested state)	6 min or as needed
Cool-down	N/A	5 min

Designing Advanced Training Programs

It is suggested that the following key areas are of greatest concern when designing an advanced training program: repetition intensity and duration, work-to-rest ratio, total exercise volume, training frequency, load, and training progression (Plisk, 1991). Intensity can be provided by training to momentary muscle failure while ensuring that the overall exercise training volume is adequate enough to create muscular and systemic overload. The work-to-rest (exercise-to-relief) ratio allows for enough recovery for the group to move with good technique. This also means that program design and exercise order play a significant role in the success of your group, as well as ensure injury prevention. Alternating upper- and lower-body exercises is an effective method to ensure adequate recovery while still providing sufficient intensity.

Repetition Intensity and Duration

Exercise intensity is the primary stimulus for HIIT and MT. Anaerobic energy pathways are best trained with shorter exercises that emphasize intensity or speed (without compromising technique) rather than with longer duration aerobic endurance exercise. The focus should be on exercise quality, not quantity, and sufficient intensity for eliciting optimal training responses and adaptations (Plisk, 1991). Good movement quality is the key for providing safe and effective workouts for your groups.

Work-to-Rest Ratio

Recovery is of significant concern during HIIT and MT workouts because phosphocreatine is the most rapid supplier of ATP for the contracting muscle proteins (Girard, Mendez-Villaneuva, & Bishop, 2011). It can take up to three minutes for complete phosphocreatine resynthesis after a bout. Experts suggest beginning with a 1-to-4 work-to-rest ratio and then, over a period of weeks, tapering to a 1-to-2 or 1-to-1.5 ratio (Plisk, 1991). In an SGT setting, you might perform timed sets with one minute for each exercise followed by 15 to 30 seconds for recovery in the following order: A lower-body exercise, followed by an upper-body movement, followed by a core drill, and finally a plyometric or high-intensity interval on a rower. This allows for around a 1-to-4 ratio of work to rest. In this instance, the strength training provides active recovery from the cardiovascular bout. Table 10.4 shows a simple MT circuit with 15

TABLE 10.4 Sample MT Circuit Workout

Work (60 s)	Transition (15 s)	Work (60 s)	Transition (15 s)	Work (60 s)	Transition (15 s)	Work (60 s)	Rest (60 s)
Deadlift		Push-up		Cable chop		Row or ride (all-out effort)	Passive recovery
Front lunge		Chin-up		Medicine ball Russian twist		Row or ride (all-out effort)	Passive recovery
Squat		Push press		Plank or side plank		Row or ride (all-out effort)	Passive recovery
Crossover lunge		Dumbbell row		Supine bicycle		Row or ride (all-out effort)	Passive recovery

seconds of recovery between exercises as transition time to get to and set up the next exercise. Actual recovery would be the end of the quad-set before the series would be repeated for two to three more sets.

Total Exercise Volume

Evidence-based guidelines for HIIT and MT conditioning regarding total workout volume (i.e., the total number of repetitions, sets, and circuits) have yet to be established (Kravitz, 2014 & Vella, 2004) This makes it essential that you carefully supervise your class, watching for any signs of acute excessive fatigue or chronic overtraining. Use open-ended questions before the warm-up to see how your groups are enjoying their workouts, how sore their muscles are, and to gauge their quality of sleep and recovery.

Training Frequency

It is suggested that trained individuals take two to three rest days per week, allowing for sufficient recovery between workouts to prevent overtraining (Plisk, 1991). With the sympathetic system in overdrive, elevated resting heart rate, poor sleep quality, and mood disturbances may occur. By allowing the body to fully recover, it permits the parasympathetic and sympathetic nervous system to find a better balance. If people are reporting poor sleep quality, irritability, unexplained weight loss, or higher resting heart rate, a few days of rest would be recommended.

Load

Resistance training that includes a high metabolic load—sets of 10 to 20 repetitions maximum—have proved most optimal (Girard et al., 2011). This is good news for timed circuit training formats: A one-minute station will allow for 15 to 20 well-performed repetitions. It is also recommended that resistance training involve controlled eccentric contractions, again with optimal technique being the goal (Plisk, 1991). This also means that the timing of the rep is important; recent studies have demonstrated that the eccentric contraction has the greatest impact on muscle hypertrophy.

Training Progression

Periodized training is considered a superior method of training for developing peak performance in athletes (Turner 2011). Due to individual goals and differences within the group, SGT instructors need to be concerned with finding the ideal training stimulus while avoiding overtraining (Plisk, 1991). Through careful consideration of the group's fitness levels, training experience, and goals, the optimal program can provide the ideal amount of intensity and volume without the threat of overtraining or injury.

Benefits of Advanced Training Programs

A comprehensive research review on HIIT reports that healthy adults can improve cardiorespiratory fitness ($\dot{V}O_2$max) 4 to 46 percent in training periods lasting 2 to 15 weeks (Boutcher, 2011). Other studies add that HIIT appears to provide rapid changes in $\dot{V}O_2$max (Kravitz, 2014 & Vella, 2004). The most recent scientific explanation for this improvement in $\dot{V}O_2$max is that HIIT causes an increase in stroke volume (volume of blood pumped by the heart per beat), which happens mainly because the heart muscle's contractility increases at near-maximal exertion (Boutcher, 2011).

Also, HIIT increases mitochondrial biogenesis (the size and number of mitochondria increase, allowing the cells' energy-producing organelles to make more ATP), which readily translates into improved cardiovascular capacity at any level of exercise intensity (Boutcher, 2011). Mitochondrial density can also significantly affect the body's ability to burn fat. An increase in mitochondrial density, therefore, is like increasing the size of your oven—a larger oven can bake a bigger turkey! By enhancing mitochondrial biogenesis, you are improving your body's fat-burning metabolism, potentially improving body composition and decreasing body fat percentages.

The high increase in epinephrine and norepinephrine from HIIT training may be a catalyst for improving fat loss; these fight-or-flight hormones have been shown to drive lipolysis (the breakdown of fat) and are largely responsible for the release of fat from both subcutaneous and intramuscular fat stores for use as fuel during exercise (Boutcher, 2011). It appears that significant changes in body weight and body fat percentage require at least 12 weeks of HIIT, which is an important factor to explain to your groups (Kessler et al., 2012). This could be a good incentive for people to continue to sign up beyond a four-week time frame.

Another highly significant benefit of HIIT is the improvement in $\dot{V}O_2$max linked to enhanced protection from heart disease (Vella, 2004). HIIT's dramatic effects on improving insulin sensitivity are also important. Additionally, the effects of HIIT on visceral and subcutaneous fat loss are encouraging.

Excess Post-Oxygen Consumption

Excess post-oxygen consumption (EPOC), or the calories expended postexercise, is often reported about in the media, with program creators making claims that the afterburn is capable of incinerating fat faster. In fact, EPOC represents the oxygen consumption above resting level that the body is utilizing to return itself to the preexercise state (Vella, 2004). The physiological mechanisms responsible for this increased metabolism (all chemical reactions in the body to liberate energy that is measured by oxygen consumption) include the replenishment of oxygen stores, phosphagen (ATP-PC) resynthesis, lactate removal, and the increased ventilation, blood circulation, and body temperature above preexercise levels (Borsheim & Bahr, 2003).

Studies demonstrate that the magnitude (amount of elevation in oxygen consumption) and duration (length of time the oxygen consumption is elevated) of EPOC is dependent on intensity and duration of exercise. It generally takes anywhere from 15 minutes to 48 hours for the body to fully recover to a resting state. Other factors influencing EPOC include training status and sex of the client (Vella, 2004).

The intensity of a cardiovascular exercise bout has the greatest impact on EPOC. As the exercise intensity increases, the magnitude and duration of EPOC increases. This means that the higher the intensity and volume, the greater the EPOC and therefore the greater the caloric expenditure postexercise. The duration of a cardiovascular exercise bout also affects EPOC. Research consistently reports a direct relationship between the duration of exercise and

EPOC. Several studies have concluded that intermittent anaerobic exercise bouts (HIIT) elicit a greater EPOC response when compared to continuous (steady-state) aerobic exercise bouts. Additionally, incorporating high-intensity intervals into continuous exercise has also been found to significantly increase EPOC (Kaminski & Whaley, 1993).

Other Advanced Training Options

HIIT, MT, and LTT are the most common types of advanced training modalities, but there are a few other training options worth mentioning.

Peripheral Heart Action (PHA)

PHA training alternates upper-body exercises with lower-body exercises with minimum rest in between. PHA benefits include increased muscular strength and maximum oxygen consumption, along with multiple cardioprotective health benefits. This simple format can be an effective class design when strength and cardiovascular benefits are the goals (Piras, Persiani, Damiani, Perazzolo, & Raffi, 2015).

Tables 10.5 and 10.6 are two examples of different formatting for PHA workouts. The setup in table 10.5 uses repeat sets before moving to the next dual set. Here, heavier loads with few reps provide the intensity. Table 10.6 is a circuit format that uses lighter loads and higher reps to create the intensity. In this workout, stations are set up around the training area. Each exercise is performed for one minute with a 10 to 15 second transition to the next station. Once the round is completed, recover for one to two minutes before repeating the circuit for a total of two to four rounds.

TABLE 10.5 Sample PHA Training Workout: Repeat Sets

Dual set 1	a. Dumbbell front squat with goblet grip: 8-12 reps	b. Full or modified push-up: 8-12 reps	10-15 s transition
Dual set 2	a. Dumbbell alternating side lunge: 8-12 reps each side	b. Dumbbell bent-over row: 8-12 reps	10-15 s transition
Dual set 3	a. Dumbbell alternating front step-up: 8-12 reps each side	b. Dumbbell push press: 8-12 reps	10-15 s transition
Dual set 4	a. Dumbbell deadlift: 8-12 reps	b. Sword draw with resistance band: 8-12 reps	10-15 s transition
Complete each dual set for 2-3 sets, with only transitional recovery as recommended. When a dual set is completed, rest 1-2 min, then move to the next set.			

TABLE 10.6   **Sample PHA Training Workout: Circuit Style**

1. Dumbbell front squat	1 min	10-15 s transition
2. Push-up	1 min	10-15 s transition
3. Alternating side lunge	1 min	10-15 s transition
4. Bent-over row (bilateral or unilateral)	1 min	10-15 s transition
5. Front step-up	1 min	10-15 s transition
6. Push press	1 min	10-15 s transition
7. Deadlift (bilateral or unilateral)	1 min	10-15 s transition
8. Sword draw (bilateral or unilateral)	1 min	10-15 s transition
Rest 1-2 min, then repeat all exercises again for a total of 2-4 rounds.		

Superset Training

Reciprocal superset training, or simply superset training, is a method that targets opposing muscle groups with little to no rest between exercises. For example, a client may complete a set of biceps curls and immediately perform a set of triceps extensions before any recovery is taken. One of the beauties of this workout structure is that there is minimal time wasted and the clients are more or less moving continuously. This lack of downtime maintains the group energy and a higher level of focus. A study that compared superset training with traditional resistance training reported significantly greater energy expenditure with superset training than with traditional resistance training (Kelleher, Hackney, Fairchild, Keslacy, & Ploutz-Snyder, 2010). The expenditure was 8.1 kilocalories per minute versus 6.2 kilocalories per minute, as well as 33 percent higher EPOC levels at 60 minutes postexercise. The protocol involved performing a set of an agonist exercise immediately followed by performing a set of the opposing muscle actions. Each exercise was performed to maximal voluntary muscle fatigue. After each superset, the subjects had 60 seconds of recovery before moving to the next exercise.

This study has significant implications for weight-management goal-based SGT classes. With an overall higher energy expenditure and EPOC, participants get more benefit, even with the same exercises. Plus, it involves no high-impact exercises and no fast movements, making it a good option for older adults or for individuals who can't perform these types of exercises or don't like plyometrics.

The six exercises in the study performed at 70 percent of 1RM of each individual's capacity are as follows:

- Bench press
- Bent-over row
- Biceps curls
- Lying triceps extension
- Leg extension
- Leg curls

In the Trenches

Irene Lewis-McCormick, MS, CSCS, author, exercise physiologist, fitness education provider and consultant, and Orangetheory Fitness head coach, from Ames, Iowa, shares her experience with teaching HIIT in small-group training settings:

- High-intensity interval training can improve fitness and transition people to the next level of training. When designed properly, a high-intensity interval using ratios of 3-to-1, 2-to-1, or 1-to-1 will take a client across the anaerobic threshold. This translates to controlled overload. As a result, adaptations can include increased $\dot{V}O_2$max, increased insulin sensitivity, improvements in blood pressure, and decreased body fat, particularly abdominal fat.

- Teaching HIIT in smaller groups is important because once the interval starts, the coach or trainer needs to be able to focus on the movement quality—the intervals can be fast and furious, so it can be difficult for a trainer or coach to focus on movement quality in a large group. In a smaller group, the coach can watch all participants and the participants can understand the movement quality and intensity expectations.

- HIIT classes are primarily bodyweight training, but they can also be done with control on large equipment (cycle, treadmill, or elliptical trainer).

- Recent research has demonstrated that HIIT protocols can be very effective not only for the conditioned client, but also for deconditioned clients and those with risks for diabetes, cardiovascular disease, and obesity. Because these workouts are scalable, coaches can use this protocol to enhance the fitness level and anaerobic tolerance for many populations. However, because the intensity is very high, recovery is essential—not only between intervals, but also between workout sessions.

Summary

Studies clearly demonstrate that advanced training techniques are effective at enhancing health and fitness and improving body composition in a time-efficient manner. Incorporating these methods into your SGT sessions in the correct volume and intensity with the appropriate groups will guarantee results. Always consider the appropriateness of the exercises in relationship to the needs, goals, and current conditioning of your clients. Remember that multilevel teaching is a must. A good protocol is two to three advanced training sessions a week, with the balance of other activities coming from lower-intensity workouts, so for shorter class times with your stronger groups, it's a win-win. This area of fitness continues to evolve, and as exciting new research continues, professionals must apply the concepts in ways that suit the needs, goals, and current condition of each client and group. Thoughtfully match the workouts to your groups: When a program is suitable, you'll witness profound changes to your clients' wellness, health, and fitness.

Dynamic Warm-Ups and Cool-Downs

Warm-ups and cool-downs are essential to any workout. In a personal training setting, these can be reasonably simple: warm-ups might involve light-intensity work on a treadmill, elliptical machine, or stationary bike, and cool-downs may include some one-on-one stretching. However, this is a poor strategy for a small-group setting. Warm-ups set the stage not only for heating up the body but also creating an atmosphere of teamwork and fun. The warm-up should also be specific to the upcoming workout and include similar movements at slower tempos to rehearse and refine the exercises. The specificity principle reigns king when it comes to movement preparation! This chapter will help by describing a variety of different warm-ups appropriate for each type of workout. You will also find a sample warm-up routine with a good general range of movements appropriate for regular strength and conditioning.

Foam-rolling self-myofascial release techniques can be applied for most cool-down sessions, but other simple strategies include classic static stretching as well as dynamic and active stretching. Depending on the group you're working with and their needs and skills, you'll find a variety of cool-downs may suit your groups. This chapter also includes a sample cool-down routine that focuses on general key muscle stretches.

Warm-Up and Cool-Down Safety Considerations

Adequate warm-ups and cool-downs are a safety issue—preparing the body for any workout is important. More than just increasing core temperature, an effective warm-up can prepare the movement skills that will be used in the workout. Rehearsing dynamic movements at slower tempos can be valuable to anyone at the beginning of a workout—for the newbie, it provides the opportunity to learn a skill at lower intensity, and for the advanced participant, it allows them to move in planes and ranges of motion that will specifically prep them for the upcoming session. Therefore, from a safety perspective, warm-ups teach valuable mechanics before other variables such as speed, load, or volume are added. This simple strategy can help keep your participants safer through skill development.

When considering a high-intensity workout, it's easy to appreciate how an appropriate warm-up can prevent or decrease the likelihood of injury. A warmer muscle is more compliant and pliable, and the increase in core temperature also decreases synovial fluid viscosity, thereby preparing the joints as well as muscles. Furthermore, this increase in core temperature and elevation in heart rate enhances circulation and prepares the cardiovascular system for work.

An appropriate cool-down is important to decrease the likelihood of any cardiac abnormalities by allowing the heart rate to gradually descend back to resting rates. The period immediately after exercise is particularly of concern because of the high generalized vasodilation. When you combine the peripheral arterial dilation caused by exercise (vasodilation) and reduced cardiac output, resulting from suddenly stopping movement, there is a resulting diminished venous return that may lead to a reduction in coronary circulation in early recovery while the heart rate is still elevated—meaning that abruptly stopping exercise can cause dizziness, fainting, and even potential cardiac arrhythmias due to venous pooling (Fletcher et al., 2001).

Although cardiac and circulatory issues certainly warrant cool-down, recent studies suggest that it does not reduce postexercise delayed onset of muscle soreness (DOMS). Rob Herbert, a senior research fellow at Neuroscience Research Australia and senior author of a foundational study of cooling down, concluded that a "warm up performed immediately prior to unaccustomed eccentric exercise produces small reductions in DOMS but [a] cool down performed after exercise does not." Rather than reducing muscle soreness, this conclusion emphasizes the psychological benefits of a cool-down: It feels good to perform some static stretches and may enhance overall flexibility when performed while the body is still warm postworkout.

Types of Stretching

Before getting started on any specific warm-up or cool-down, some definitions and applications need to be established. It's important to understand the different types of stretching appropriate for a variety of participants in an SGT class. Different methods are applicable to different phases of the workout and for diverse populations. Not every warm-up or cool-down protocol will suit all participants. The art here is in choosing the best, most appropriate stretches for the type of class and for the level of your students.

Dynamic Movement Stretching

Dynamic movement stretching involves whole-body movements, typically including functional movement patterns in all three planes of motion. These movement flows can be repeated while moving in place or back and forth across the room. This type of stretching is ideal for warm-ups, and can also be used in cool-downs when the workout has been very intense and heart rates are elevated. It is perfect for intermediate to advanced participants who have good body control, balance, and coordination, but is not recommended for extremely deconditioned individuals with poor balance or body control. Dynamic movement stretching should be performed for 5 to 10 minutes, depending on the workout.

Active Isolated Stretching

Active isolated stretching involves activating agonists to shut down tight antagonists. For example, one effective chest stretch is to hold the arms out to the side of the body at shoulder height and pull the elbows back by contracting the posterior deltoids and rhomboids (agonists) to lengthen the pectorals (antagonists). This type of stretching is not intended as whole-body integrated stretching; however, some isolated stretches can be included as part of a dynamic warm-up, as an effective cool-down, or as part of the workout. Active isolated stretching is ideally suited for most populations and can be especially helpful as part of a warm-up for less-conditioned participants, because it requires less balance and stability and is performed in more supported environments. This type of stretch can also be helpful for problem areas of the body such as the chest, shoulders, or hips. It is recommended to perform one to two sets of five or more reps, holding the end range of motion for two to five seconds.

Myofascial Release

Utilizing a foam roller or similar device, myofascial release involves rolling tight areas of the body, applying constant pressure back and forth along a small area for 30 to 45 seconds. A small ball can also be helpful for smaller or tighter areas of the body. A knot or particularly uncomfortable section of rolling typically represents muscle fibers that are not in alignment; rolling can therefore help relax and align fibers in the direction of healthy muscles. Rolling can be performed as part of a warm-up routine for more strength-related training, or as part of a cool-down.

This technique is particularly effective for participants with postural imbalances, especially if they are sedentary. For individuals who spend large amounts of time seated, you can expect the hips, hamstrings, and thoracic spine to be tight. Tight hips, especially the psoas, can also contribute to tightness in the ankles. If this is the case, starting from the lower extremities and moving up the body is a good strategy.

If you're short on time, start with the calf, move to the hips, and then move up the back to the thoracic spine. It's typical to find small areas of the body where the release is more intense. When this is the case, stop and hold the position and focus on breathing. If, for example, there's a spot on the calf that feels significant, hold with as much pressure as possible and circle the ankle. If the tender spot is on the quadriceps or IT band, try bending and straightening the knee while maintaining constant pressure on top of the knot.

Static Passive Stretching

Static passive stretching is muscle specific and not intended as a whole-body, integrated focus. Static passive stretching is ideal for the end of a cool-down when the goal is to improve flexibility. Static stretching should not be used as a warm-up and should only be used on muscles that are already well warmed up. First, static stretching is a suboptimal method to increase total-body circulation and heat. Once you've adequately warmed up the body, muscles are more pliable. There is some controversy surrounding stretching as part of a warm-up, particularly if the workout to follow is high intensity, in which case stretching may actually inhibit the ability to achieve full intensity (Simic, Sarabon, & Markovic, 2013). This inhibition is attributed to the fact that stretching improves muscle elasticity by decreasing muscle viscosity, thereby lowering the force-generating capacity of the contractile proteins of the muscle. If the goal of the group is to improve flexibility, static stretching can be performed after an effective warm-up has been implemented.

Static stretching is suitable for all populations and does not require any special skills or abilities; many of the stretches can be performed supine, side lying, or standing. Perform two to four reps held for 15 to 30 seconds each and target major muscle groups. It is important to note that at around five seconds of stretch tension, individuals may experience a burning sensation. If this occurs, move out of the stretch, relax a moment, and then move back into the position. If shaking occurs at the end range of the stretch, decrease range of motion until the shaking stops to prevent injury. The stretches should feel pleasant and held to a mild, comfortable point of tension.

Dynamic Warm-Up

When examining what constitutes an effective warm-up, it's important to consider what you are trying to achieve and the type of class that's going to follow. Mental and physical readiness, injury prevention, and performance enhancement are the main objectives in movement preparation. Warm-ups have evolved from traditional static stretching to a more dynamic approach. Recent studies demonstrate that holding static stretches slows down neural messaging, does not decrease the rate of injury, and can even inhibit muscular performance. One study looked at a total of 104 previous studies on stretching and athletic performance and found that, regardless of age, sex, or fitness level, static stretching before a workout impaired explosive movement and strength performance (Simic et al., 2013). Simic's study revealed that the duration of the stretch created pronounced decreases in isometric and dynamic strength production that were not related to age, sex, or fitness level. It was discovered that the smallest negative acute effects were observed with stretch duration equal to or greater than 45 seconds. The study confirmed that the use of static stretching as the sole warm-up activity should generally be avoided. In another study on the acute effects of static stretching on muscle strength and power, the antiperformance effects of preworkout static stretching is illustrated clearly. (Chaabene et al., 2019). Although more research is needed into the exact mechanism of why static stretching hurts performance so much, it is believed that that loosening muscles and tendons by a traditional manner leaves individuals less able to move quickly and on command.

A dynamic warm-up can increase blood flow and core temperature and, as mentioned, potentially disrupt temporary connective tissue bonds, with the following effects on performance:

- Faster muscle contraction and relaxation of both agonist and antagonist muscles
- Improvements in rate of force development
- Improvements in reaction time
- Improvements in muscle strength and power

- Lowered viscous resistance in muscles
- Increased blood flow to active muscles
- Enhanced metabolic reactions

Warm-ups also provide a rehearsal of upcoming movements, allowing your class an opportunity to learn basic exercises at slower speeds and lower intensities. Energetically speaking, a good warm-up builds atmosphere and team bonding. It's a time for you to connect with your group and each individual with eye contact, enthusiasm, and a bright smile!

A dynamic stretching routine is standard for athletes ranging from amateurs to professionals. As the term implies, a dynamic warm-up uses stretches that are movement based rather than static. This is ideal for many reasons:

- It activates the muscles you will specifically use during your workout at a lower intensity, providing an opportunity to instruct technique and rehearse the movement.
- Dynamic stretches can help you feel more limber and loosen up tighter areas of the body (Page, 2012).
- Dynamic stretching improves body awareness because it involves whole-body exercise drills that challenge coordination, balance, and movement skills.
- Motion-based warm-ups have been demonstrated to enhance muscular performance and power (Beedle & Mann, 2007).

The length and intensity of a warm-up is dependent on a number of factors, including the ambient temperature, the time of the day, the age of your group, and the intensity of the work to be performed (a higher-intensity workout necessitates a longer and more vigorous warm-up). Older populations may also need a longer but less intense warm-up, whereas cold-weather and early-morning workouts will also need longer warm-ups but of greater intensity.

A dynamic warm-up duration can be anything between 5 and 10 minutes. The movement selection should consist of all primary movement patterns (bilateral bend and lift, single leg, push, pull, and rotate) in all three planes of motion. It's also essential to consider the types of movement patterns that will be performed in the workout itself, as well as the skill level of the participants. Simplicity is golden, especially with less-coordinated groups with balance challenges. Remember, the warm-up not only sets the physical stage, but also the psychological state, so it's critical that your group feels successful.

For your dynamic warm-up, create around 8 to 10 reps of each exercise for 1 to 2 rounds, like a circuit. Focus on good quality movement and posture to set the expectation for the upcoming workout. There are three basic approaches depending on your space, group size, and the age or skill level of your group: Rehearsal movements of the upcoming exercises performed at low intensity, traveling line drills, or on-the-spot movement. There are advantages and disadvantages to each.

Rehearsal movements are good for machine-based training where there's not a lot of open space. In this case, participants do one set (rotation) of each station. Then, from the second set on, they increase the load, speed, or intensity of the station. This method is very space efficient, it's a great warm-up for circuit training workouts, and participants can master or improve their skills at a lower intensity.

Traveling line drills involve moving back and forth in lines performing each exercise. This warm-up is more dynamic, thereby increasing core temperature more rapidly and establishing a flow. However, it requires significantly more space, the balance and coordination challenges are increased, and it is harder to teach in larger groups.

The on-the-spot movement drills comprise many of the same exercises as line drills, except they are performed in place. This is an advantage for visual learners because you typically warm up with them, giving them an opportunity to watch and follow. This type of warm-up is also space efficient, typically only requiring each person's arm width, squared. The other advantage is that these movements typically require less balance and coordination, making them good for newer, less skilled clients. The disadvantage to this warm-up is that it is less dynamic, so you may need a little longer to get your group warmed up adequately, especially if you are going to be working out at higher intensities.

The five moves in the following sample warm-up provide a great on-the-spot total-body dynamic warm-up that moves through all three planes of motion and is suitable for most workout formats and most participants. Perform each exercise for one minute. For the unilateral movements such as the hip circle and side lunge with arm sweep, perform each side for 60 seconds. With transitions and demonstrations, the total warm-up time is around seven minutes.

Sample Total-Body Dynamic Warm-Up

1. Hip Hinge

Stand with feet hip width apart. Hinge forward at the hip while keeping knees soft and feel a light stretch in the hamstrings (see figure *a*). Stand up and open the front body, reaching arms overhead and driving hips forward (see figure *b*).

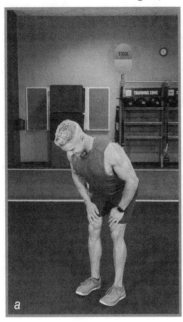
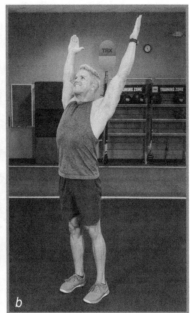

2. Squat, Cat-Cow, Punch, and Rotate

Start by standing with feet hip width apart and toes forward. Squat down (see figure *a*), then round up like an angry cat with hands on thighs (see figure *b*). Squat down again (see figure *c*), then stand up to punch across the body and rotate body to the same side (see figure *d*).

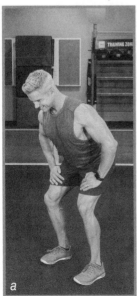
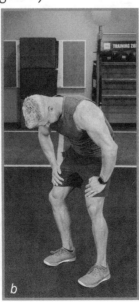
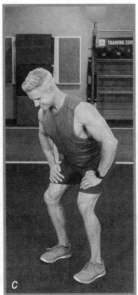
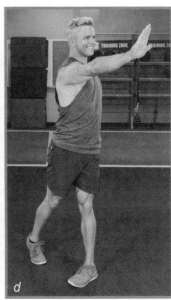

3. Front Lunge and Lean

Start by standing with feet together. Step forward with the left leg, bending both knees into a lunge. Reach the hands overhead (see figure *a*) and lean the body to the right side, reaching high (see figure *b*). Come back to center and alternate sides.

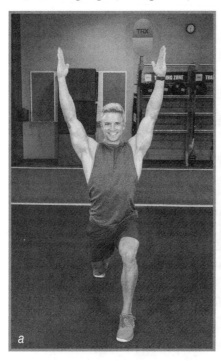
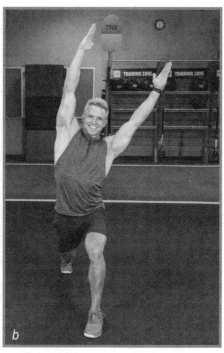

4. Hip Circle and Side Lunge With Arm Sweep

Start by standing with feet together. Stand on the left leg and perform a hip circle with the right leg (see figure *a*). Then, keeping feet parallel, lunge to the right, bending the right knee while extending the left and sweep arms across the body to the right, rotating the whole upper body (see figure *b*). Repeat all repetitions on one side before performing the exercise on the other side.

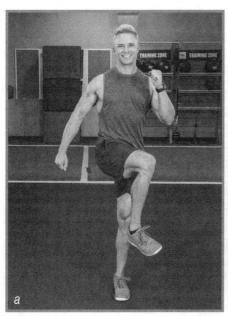
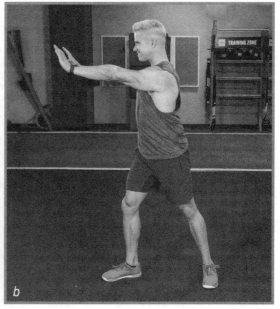

5. Plank Walk-Down and Push-Up With Body Rock

Begin in a forearm plank (see figure *a*). Walk hands up to a high plank (see figure *b*) and do a push-up. Next, bend both knees, rocking hips back toward the heels, flexing the shoulders and lowering the upper body towards the floor as the hips rock back and upward (see figure *c*). Finally, walk hands down to the forearm plank position.

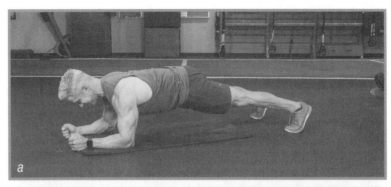

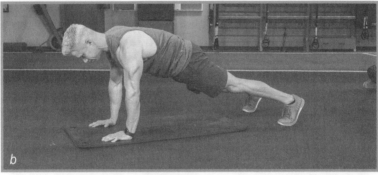

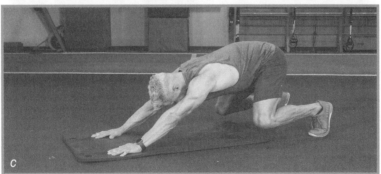

Effective Cool-Downs

Because stopping exercise abruptly can cause blood to pool in the lower extremities, leading to dizziness or fainting, an effective cool-down is important. Simply by keeping the legs moving at the end of a workout with walking or similar low-intensity activity, you can maintain normal circulation to the brain. This is especially important when the class has centered on high-intensity interval training (HIIT). If heart rate is high at the end of the workout, dynamic movement stretching performed slowly is a good strategy. This can include hip circles, side-to-side bodyweight lunges, overhead reaches, and shoulder circles or arm circles. Similarly to warm-ups, these can be done as traveling line drills or in one spot. When strength and muscular endurance is the focus and heart rate is not high at the end, transitioning into dynamic and eventually to static and passive stretching is a good plan.

Regular flexibility training is an important component of a comprehensive fitness program and should be included in your SGT classes. Flexibility refers to the degree of tissue extensibility around a joint that allows for a functional range of motion. It is dependent on muscle properties and the nervous system's ability to efficiently control movement throughout the range of motion. Individual differences in joint structure, age, and previous injury all affect flexibility.

Whether the goal is to improve range of motion, improve mental state, or relax and assist in cooling the body down, some form of regular stretching is one of the keys to overall well-being. There are numerous benefits associated with good flexibility, including improved posture, increased range of motion, restored muscle balance, reduced joint stress, and improved movement efficiency. Training for flexibility could even be a full program with these specific goals. Many trainers run SGT classes that focus exclusively on flexibility, as well as yoga and Pilates groups.

Leaving 5 to 10 minutes at the end of your classes to allow time to stretch is a good habit. The following sample cool-down covers most muscles while focusing on key muscles that have a tendency to be tight and cause joint imbalances, especially at the hips and shoulders. Hold each stretch for 15 to 30 seconds and move slowly to promote a feeling of relaxation. Repeat each stretch if you have a bit more time. Breath slowly and smoothly throughout each stretch.

Sample Floor-Based Static Stretch Cool-Down

1. Supine Lower Back Stretch

Lie on your back and pull both knees into the chest, allowing your tailbone to curl off the floor. Take a deep breath into your lower belly and feel the expansion of your lower back.

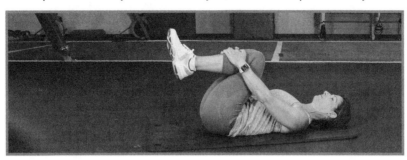

2. Supine Hip Stretch

Lie on your back and pull one knee into the chest while extending the other leg along the floor with the knee straight. Work to keep the straight leg on the floor as much as possible while feeling a stretch in the back of the hip and thigh in the bent leg and the front of the hip in the straight leg.

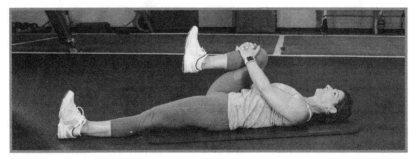

3. Supine Hamstring and Active Calf Stretch

Lie on your back and extend one knee, holding the other leg at the hamstring or calf. Flex the foot to actively stretch the calf. As you straighten the leg toward the ceiling, push up through your heel to emphasize the stretch in both the calf and hamstring.

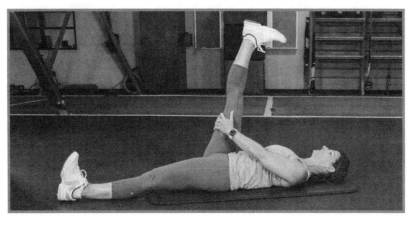

4. Supine Figure 4 Hip Stretch

Lying on your back, cross ankle over thigh with your open knee to the side, like a figure 4 shape. Pull the other knee to chest while trying to open the knee of the hip being stretched. To further increase the stretch, perform a small circular motion of the held leg, and work with deep, slow, gentle breathing. Repeat the whole sequence on the other side.

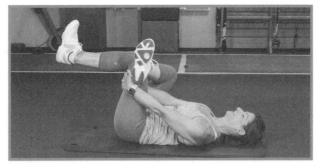

5. Spinal Roll

Lie on your back and pull both knees to chest. Roll forward and back on the spine while staying off the neck. Gradually increase the amplitude of the rocking and add a little balance on the sit bones at the top of the movement.

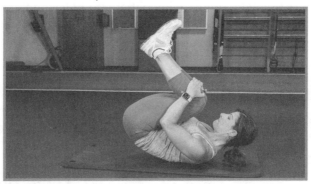

6. Side-Body Stretch

Sitting cross-legged and keeping both sit bones on the floor, reach one arm up overhead and lean to the opposite side, stretching the side of the body. Inhale as you reach up and exhale as you lean to the side, feeling the length between the hip and tip of the fingers.

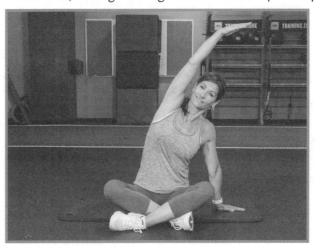

7. Triceps Stretch

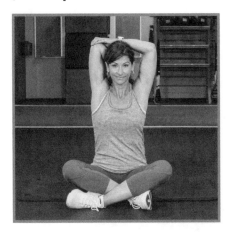

Sitting cross-legged, extend one arm over the head, reaching hand down between the shoulder blades (as if patting your own back). Gently press the elbow with the opposite hand to deepen the stretch. To further increase the stretch, press the elbow back and lift chin to look forward. Use the exhalation to assist in the feeling of relaxation.

8. Rear Shoulder Stretch

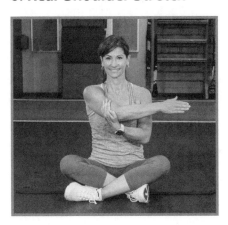

Sitting cross-legged, bring the arm across the chest, keeping the shoulder down, away from the ear. Holding the arm above the elbow with the other hand, gently press toward the chest, stretching the back of the shoulder.

9. Spinal Twist

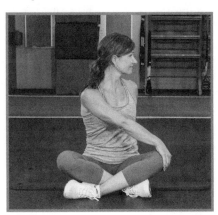

Sit cross-legged and hold the left knee with the right hand, reaching the left hand onto the floor behind, rotating the spine. Look behind, with the head following in the direction of the stretch. Alternate sides.

10. Side-Lying Quad and Hip Stretch

Lie on your side, resting on your elbow and forearm. Take the foot of the top leg with the same-side hand and gently pull the foot toward the buttocks while pressing the hips forward, rotating the pelvis under, holding the knees close together.

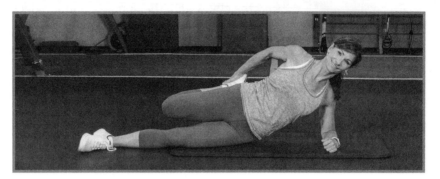

In the Trenches

Gina De Roma, C-IAYT, E-RYT-200, CMP, KSM, a certified yoga therapist and state-certified massage therapist with over 17 years of experience, teaches small-group training classes and corporate wellness in Los Angeles. De Roma travels to homes and offices and other workplace settings to train her small groups.

De Roma believes that flexibility is key to the health and performance of both body and mind. According to De Roma, "our muscles need both compacting and lengthening exercises in order to provide the flexibility that helps prevent injury. Our spines need more opportunities to put some space between the vertebrae, as nearly everything we do in our modern world (walking, sitting, commuting, hunching over devices) compacts the spine. Flexibility of mind is equally important to our well-being, as our modern technology and social media can overload the brain with too much information. Taking even a few moments a day for emptying the mind with visualization or guided meditation is key to reducing stress and improving mental performance, just as taking time to stretch the body is key to physical well-being and fitness."

De Roma's warm-ups vary, as do the yoga flows themselves, depending on the client or group. For example, De Roma trains one older couple three times a week who had never practiced yoga prior to working with her. According to De Roma, now they are enthusiastically moving through a full Ashtanga/power yoga–style flow. She explains, "on those days I will warm-up with quite a bit of hip-opening poses to protect the knees during all of the sun-salutations."

She continues, "One thing that never varies is that we begin each and every yoga session with the breath; deep, conscious breathing that completely fills and empties the lungs." For De Roma, the breath is the foundation of any and every yoga practice. "Focusing on the breath helps keep us focused on the moment and out of our egos, which helps to prevent injury as well."

In corporate settings, De Roma has found that "some of my most rewarding teaching experiences have been within a corporate setting. I love seeing the shift in attitude on an employee's face after a few minutes of chair yoga or guided meditation. I once spoke to a group of hospice volunteers at Kaiser about self-care and was able to share the story of my dad's cancer battle and how small acts of kindness can have healing effects well beyond our immediate awareness. Sharing the power of making a difference uplifted me as well as the group I was speaking to."

Summary

Like bookends, warm beginnings and cool endings frame your sessions and keep your classes safer and more effective. Remember to consider the demands the workout will place on your groups and provide a warm-up that prepares for those stresses. If that session is going to be high intensity, then gradually increase heart rate and core temperature to harder levels of work without creating initial fatigue. If the session involves free-standing exercises, then incorporating whole-body, three-dimensional movements through multiple planes is a winning choice. By using specific strategies for warm-ups, you'll initiate your classes with optimal movements that better prepare your clients for the upcoming workout.

From a similar perspective, cool-downs should also be specific—not just to the workout, but also for the time of the day. For example, after a morning session, it may be better to perform a "lively" cool-down to prepare people to move into their day. In the evening, a more calming and relaxing stretch will leave your groups feeling soothed and peaceful for an optimal night's sleep.

As with every consideration for your group, be conscious of their needs, goals, and current condition to ensure you're providing the best possible practices for your warm-ups and cool-downs.

PART IV

SAMPLE PROGRAMS

CHAPTER 12

Introductory Training Programs

The programs in this chapter are designed to be less intense and more suitable for the newer, deconditioned participant. A less challenging workout is a good approach, especially those with lower self-efficacy; they will manage the workout well and finish feeling successful.

If you've done a full evaluation of your clients and grouped those with similar fitness levels, this group is likely to be, at the very least, in the early action stages of change. This means that they've only been working out regularly for a few months and may have had several prior unsuccessful attempts at training. This is why it's so critical that these initial workouts be doable. Remember, one of your primary goals as an instructor is to help your clients become lifelong exercisers. They are at the beginning stages of making that happen with you as their guide. Typically, these folks have been working out for one to six months and are still prone to dropping out. Every tool for retention is critical, and one of the main tools is to keep the workouts fun and easy. By keeping the exercises simple, the loads light, and workouts easy to navigate, new participants can build not only fitness, but also self-efficacy and confidence.

Note that the third program described in this chapter, the Functional Active and Aging Workout, is for the active older adult. Although this heterogeneous group may or may not be deconditioned, it's included here with the lower-intensity workouts and could be utilized for individuals of any age who are in poor physical condition—for example, a sedentary 40-year-old who hasn't done any exercise in over a year. Whether you're working with active older adults or deconditioned middle-aged groups, these programs are low impact and do not include jumping, explosive movement, or power training, which makes them a good starting point to ease into an active lifestyle.

Simple Circuit Workout

This program is designed to improve muscular strength endurance as well as cardiovascular fitness. Because you move from lower-body to upper-body exercise for a full circuit with minimal rest, the cardiovascular demand increases heart rate, thereby enhancing fitness. To achieve this training effect, it is critical to take minimal recovery between exercises, using only necessary transitional time. This simple Peripheral Heart Action (PHA) circuit is modified to suit less-conditioned participants. PHA can be adapted to all populations by a manipulation of the energy demands of each movement (complexity and intensity) and the amount of time used to transition between the exercises. Other variables, such as speed of movement, integration of body parts, recovery, repetitions, and load, all affect intensity. If you're looking to progress or regress this program, choose one or more of these variables to achieve the goal.

Although this workout maintains cardiovascular intensity with minimal recovery intervals, the exercises are simple and easy to master. These recovery times can easily be extended to accommodate less-conditioned folks, keeping in mind that the overall intensity and cardiovascular demands of the workout are somewhat dependent on the transition time between exercises—the longer the interexercise recovery, the less cardiovascular intensity. You may also consider beginning with shorter workouts, longer warm-ups, increased postexercise stretching, and keeping the interexercise recovery shorter. This can accomplish enough to get your participants on the road to becoming more active. Keep in mind, deconditioned individuals will do better with less! With less duration, intensity, or load, they will experience less muscle soreness and greater self-confidence. As with any exercise program, you can manipulate the training variables to suit the needs of your participants. Whether you shorten the overall work by lengthening the warm-up and cool-down, or lengthen the interexercise recovery to decrease intensity (if needed), you can make this work for your group accordingly.

SETUP AND GUIDELINES

Stations can be set up with equipment around the room, or it can be taught with everyone working simultaneously. However, for the simultaneous workout you will need more equipment and space, so the traditional circuit is better for a small space or larger group.

Perform 8 to 12 reps, choosing a load that fatigues the muscles. Complete one set of each exercise and move to the next exercise with minimal rest, performing all 10 exercises consecutively, then recover for one to two minutes. Repeat for two to three sets, depending on how much time you have to train and the experience of your clients. Transition time between each exercise is 10 to 15 seconds, resting only enough to move from one exercise and set up the next. If participants are struggling with the workout, adding more time to transition (20-30 seconds) is an excellent way to modify the session.

DURATION

45 to 60 minutes

NUMBER OF PARTICIPANTS

4 to 6

EQUIPMENT

Dumbbells, high step, cable or resistance bands, stability ball

ADDITIONAL WORKOUT NOTES

- Allow 5 to 7 minutes of dynamic total-body movements to prepare for the workout. You might try the Sample Total-Body Dynamic Warm-Up outlined in chapter 11; however, if coordination and body control are of particular concern, break the movements down further into single components. For example, the squat, cat-cow, and punch and rotate could be taught first as a squat, then as a squat with a cat-cow, then a rotational side-to-side reach, with the last step being all three movements put together. Take your time teaching this warm-up by slowing down all movements and breaking down each progression to ensure mastery.

- Increase load and range of motion (ROM) as the body adapts. Start with 8 to 12 reps to fatigue. Once this is no longer challenging, increase the reps to 15. When 15 reps are no longer challenging, increase the load until 8 to 10 reps can be performed with good technique. Utilizing a timer is another option for this workout. Set the timer for 30-45 seconds with 10-15 seconds of interexercise recovery and 60 seconds of interset rest.

- At the completion of the workout, be sure to provide your class with plenty of time to cool down. This is a great opportunity to improve flexibility and develop good stretching habits (see Sample Floor-Based Static Stretch Cool-Down, chapter 11).

Exercise	Reps/time/sets	Adaptations
Dumbbell squat	8-15 reps or 30-45 s for 1-3 sets	To regress, adjust the ROM and work in a pain-free range with the lightest dumbbell until movement can be performed with heavier load and greater range.
Cable or resistance band row	8-15 reps or 30-45 s for 1-3 sets	Choose a weight that allows full ROM while bringing the hand back to the ribcage.
Dumbbell lateral lunge (Page 190)	8-15 reps or 30-45 s for 1-3 sets	To regress, adjust the ROM and work in a pain-free range with the lightest dumbbell until movement can be performed with heavier load and greater range.
Kettlebell push press (Page 216)	8-15 reps or 30-45 s for 1-3 sets	A push press allows the client to choose a heavier weight than a strict overhead press. Make sure the client has adequate shoulder mobility and scapular and core stability to press overhead.

(continued)

Simple Circuit Workout *(continued)*

Exercise	Reps/time/sets	Adaptations
Dumbbell lateral step-up	8-15 reps or 30-45 s for 1-3 sets	The height of the step directly affects the intensity of the exercise and is dictated by the strength, fitness, and height of the client. Choose a height that places the knee at approximately 90 degrees of flexion. Work in a less aggressive ROM if the client is less conditioned, regardless of their height.
Dumbbell and stability ball chest press	8-15 reps or 30-45 s for 1-3 sets	To regress, simultaneously press the dumbbells and use a stable surface such as a weight bench instead of a ball. To progress, alternate lowering one hand at a time.
Dumbbell transverse lunge	8-15 reps or 30-45 s for 1-3 sets	To regress, adjust the ROM and work in a pain-free range with the lightest dumbbell until movement can be performed with heavier load and greater range. Hip mobility will be the limiting factor when it comes to the ROM of the movement. Work with the greatest ROM possible.
Dumbbell and stability ball supine triceps press	8-15 reps or 30-45 s for 1-3 sets	To regress this exercise, use a mat or a weight bench to provide a more stable surface.
Dumbbell deadlift	8-15 reps or 30-45 s for 1-3 sets	Ensure great technique before adding heavy load to this exercise. Do not load heavily if the client lacks hip mobility and core stability.
Dumbbell and stability ball seated biceps curl	8-15 reps or 30-45 s for 1-3 sets	To regress, sit on a stable surface. To progress, stand on an unstable surface, such as a BOSU Balance Trainer.

Posture Perfect Workout

This workout was created to help improve total-body alignment and correct typical postural imbalances common to a sedentary lifestyle. This workout focuses on strengthening the body's posterior chain and opening the anterior body through increased mobility at the hip, thoracic spine, and shoulder. Additionally, lumbar stability is addressed with various planks and bridges.

SETUP AND GUIDELINES

This workout is performed circuit style, with three mini-circuits of six different exercises per series. Time or repetitions can be used to create training volume. For time, each station should be 45 to 60 seconds; for repetitions, keep them between 12 and 15. Take 15 to 30 seconds between exercises and a full minute between sets. If you're doing multiple sets, perform each mini-circuit for those sets before moving to the next exercise series.

DURATION

30 to 45 minutes

NUMBER OF PARTICIPANTS

4 to 6

EQUIPMENT

Suspension training system, stability ball, mats (for cushioning), resistance bands (either with anchor or with teammates working in pairs)

ADDITIONAL WORKOUT NOTES

Before starting, allow 5 to 10 minutes of warm-up using the Sample Total-Body Dynamic Warm-Up outlined in chapter 11 to adequately prepare the body, loosen tight muscles, and activate the core. Also, self-myofascial release, or foam rolling, can also be an effective warm-up method for this program because this type of preparation can assist in bringing the postural muscles into a more neutral position while also increasing circulation (see chapter 11 for more on self-myofascial release).

Each exercise should be performed slowly through a full range of motion, emphasizing body control with perfect posture and alignment.

At the completion of the workout, be sure to provide your class with plenty of time to cool down. This is a great opportunity to improve flexibility and develop good stretching habits (see Sample Floor-Based Static Stretch Cool-Down, chapter 11). Foam rolling is also a good option for the end of the workout, especially focusing on creating mobility in the thoracic spine, hips, and lower legs.

Mini-circuit series 1	
Exercise	**Adaptations**
Suspension pull	To regress, move feet further away from the anchor point. To progress, move further forward under the suspension trainer.
Stability ball bridge	To progress, take two small steps to the right, allowing the right shoulder to exit the ball. Hold shoulders and hips level. Repeat left. Move slowly!
Resistance band sword draw (partner or solo if anchored) (Page 181)	To progress, try a heavier resistance band or stand further away from the attachment point.
Stability ball back extension	To progress, hold a dumbbell or reach arms overhead to lengthen the lever.
Resistance band triceps walk-back draw (partner or solo if anchored) (Page 182)	To progress, try a heavier resistance band or stand further away from the attachment point.
Bodyweight plank or side plank (Page 183)	To regress, leave knees on the floor. To progress, lift top foot off the ground into a star position.
Mini-circuit series 2	
Exercise	**Adaptations**
Suspension I-Y-W-T (Page 184)	To regress, stand more upright. To progress, stand further forward and increase body incline
Stability ball hamstring curl (Page 185)	To regress, lower hips toward the mat. To progress, try this unilaterally.
Resistance band external rotation draw (partner or solo if anchored)	To progress, try a heavier resistance band or stand further away from the attachment point.

(continued)

Posture Perfect Workout   *(continued)*

| Mini-circuit series 2 *(continued)* ||
Exercise	**Adaptations**
Stability ball plank (Page 186)	To regress, keep knees on the mat. To progress, pull elbows in and out.
Resistance band rear fly draw (partner or solo if anchored)	To progress, try a heavier resistance band or stand further away from the attachment point.
Bodyweight bridge	To progress, perform unilaterally. Pull one knee into the chest while working the other leg. Repeat on other side.
Mini-circuit series 3	
Exercise	**Adaptations**
Suspension crossover lunge and pull (Page 187)	To regress, use arms to assist more to decrease the amount of work in the legs. To progress, use arms less to create a greater challenge for the lower body.
Stability ball push-up	To regress, keep the ball under the thighs. To progress, walk out until just your feet are on the ball.
Resistance band isometric rotator cuff lateral step-out (partner or solo if anchored)	To progress, try a heavier resistance band or stand further away from the attachment point.
Stability ball I-Y-W-T	To regress, rest between reps. To progress, hold light dumbbells.
Resistance band lunge and bow and arrow (partner or solo if anchored) (Page 189)	To progress, try a heavier resistance band or stand further away from the attachment point.
Bodyweight plank with hip rotation (Page 189)	To regress, lower knees to the mat between repetitions. To progress, move very slowly between positions.

Functional Active and Aging Workout

The term *older adult* refers to individuals aged 65 and older, as well as those aged 50 to 64 with clinically significant conditions or physical limitations that affect movement, physical fitness, or physical activity. This represents a diverse spectrum of ages and physiologic capabilities (ACSM, 2017). Beyond the age of 50, there is a tendency for older individuals to lose muscle mass (sarcopenia). This is especially pronounced in women, who do not have enough testosterone to support the muscle mass (ACE, 2014). That being said, the active aging exerciser is a great market to tap into. The older adult often enjoys the social element of group training, but often needs more attention and specificity than a younger participant, and the price point of small-group training is better than personal training for those on a fixed income.

In older individuals, there are four overriding considerations that dictate modification of the exercise program (Foster et al., 2007):

1. Avoiding cardiovascular risk and being familiar with medications that can affect injury or heart rate, such as blood thinners or beta blockers

2. Avoiding orthopedic risk and being aware of any joint replacements

3. Preserving muscle tissue, especially in females

4. Recognizing the slower rate at which older individuals adapt to training

Other considerations must be made for this population: Hearing can be a challenge when working with older adults, so speak clearly and keep music appropriate with the volume adjusted so your group can hear you easily. Keep the room well-lit and the floor clear of clutter to decrease the risk of falls. Most importantly, make sure you're familiar with all the health and wellness issues your individuals may be challenged by and ensure they have medical clearance to exercise.

SETUP AND GUIDELINES

This workout is performed as a whole group rather than as a circuit and can be done either for time or reps. If you're using a timer, try 45 to 60 seconds per exercise and 15- to 30-second recovery intervals, adjusting as needed. For reps, perform 12 to 15 repetitions of each exercise with the same rest and recovery ratios mentioned previously. Complete the series of four exercises for the intended number of sets before moving to the next series.

Note that this program includes some partner training. This adds a social element while providing an external anchor point for each person when using resistance bands. If you have an uneven number of participants, you can attach the bands to a machine and have one person work solo.

DURATION

45 to 60 minutes

NUMBER OF PARTICIPANTS

4 to 6

EQUIPMENT

Dumbbells, chair, resistance bands, step platform

ADDITIONAL WORKOUT NOTES

- Allow 7 to 10 minutes of dynamic total-body movements to prepare for the workout. You might try the Sample Total-Body Dynamic Warm-Up outlined in chapter 11. This should be done at a controlled tempo with a focus on quality movement rather than speed. Break movements down into single components if coordination and balance are an issue. As your group progresses and movement quality improves, the speed and complexity of the warm-up exercises can increase.

- Older adults can vary greatly in their capacity to move. Try to group clients of similar age, fitness, and capacity. This will make it easier for you to teach and helps build camaraderie. Spend time breaking down the exercises into parts (see teaching techniques outlined in chapter 7).

- Remember that this population needs longer to learn and more time to adapt. Keep the exercises the same for six to eight weeks. Allow longer for strength to build and provide individual modifications wherever needed.

- Demonstrate movements more slowly and pace your group more carefully than you would your younger clients, especially when performing rotational movements.

- Keep equipment in front of the mat. If you're using a chair for balance, keep the mat under the chair to reduce the risk of tripping or falling.

- At the completion of the workout, be sure to provide your class with plenty of time to cool down. This is a great opportunity to improve flexibility and develop good stretching habits (see Sample Floor-Based Static Stretch Cool-Down, chapter 11), provided they can get up and down from the floor. If stretching on a mat is not an option, try adapting the stretches to a chair or from a standing position.

Series 1	
Exercise	**Adaptations**
Dumbbell reverse lunge (Page 189)	To regress, decrease ROM, speed, tempo, and load. To progress, increase ROM, speed, tempo, and load.
Deadlift with bent-over row (Page 190)	
One-arm row	
Partner side-by-side sagittal chop (Page 191)	

Series 2	
Exercise	**Adaptations**
Squat to bench	To progress the squat to bench, choose a lower bench.
Dumbbell squat curl and press (Page 192)	
Dumbbell alternating overhead press	If overhead movements are painful, then choose a very light weight or no weight at all and simply move through the ROM.
Partner side-by-side alternating rotation (Page 192)	

Series 3	
Exercise	**Adaptations**
Dumbbell or bodyweight transverse lunge (Page 193)	To regress the transverse lunge, keep the ROM small and build gradually.
Dumbbell step-up with biceps curl (Page 193)	To progress the step-up, try a higher step and heavier dumbbells.
Dumbbell biceps curl	Keep the rotation slow and controlled on the golf chop.
Dumbbell golf chop (Page 194)	

Series 4	
Exercise	**Adaptations**
Dumbbell or bodyweight bridge	If your participants cannot go to the floor, try using a step.
Dumbbell supine bridge and pullover (Page 195)	
Dumbbell supine triceps press	
Bird dog (Page 196)	If your participant has pain while kneeling for the bird dog, try padding the under the knees or perform the exercise over a stability ball.

CHAPTER 13

Advanced Training Programs

This chapter includes six advanced high-intensity metabolic training (MET) and high-intensity interval training (HIIT) programs designed for functional strength gains, hypertrophy, enhanced balance and coordination, maximum caloric expenditure, and cardiovascular conditioning. These programs are ideal for clients who already have built a good solid foundation of fitness and are looking for a challenge that will further improve cardiovascular fitness, anaerobic power, and body composition. Keep in mind that these programs would not be recommended for new, deconditioned individuals.

One of the main advantages of high-intensity training lies in the rapid fitness gains. It has been found that healthy adults can improve cardiorespiratory fitness by 4 to 46 percent in training periods lasting 2 to 15 weeks (Boutcher, 2011). At the same time, it is highly effective at helping clients improve body composition with only 12 weeks of training (Kessler, Sisson, & Short, 2012).

These metabolic and HIIT workouts are suitable for four to six participants, depending on your space and equipment availability. The equipment suggested here is specialized, but other options could also be substituted. For example, if a rower is not available, then a treadmill, stair climber, or bike could be good alternatives. Using the treadmill at an incline of 7 to 9 percent is a good way to provide intensity for walkers, whereas running intervals would work well for participants who enjoy running.

Because these workouts are high intensity, make sure you allow adequate time for warm-up and cool-down. Decreasing the length of work time and increasing the recovery intervals is a good way to introduce the programs, ensuring a good experience for everyone.

Super Circuit Workout

Like all the advanced programs described in this chapter, this workout is excellent for a group that already has great general fitness and wants to improve body composition. The Super Circuit Workout moves fast! With this HIIT workout, you'll be combining rowing or running with the use of various pieces of equipment. All of the moves are physically demanding and combining them makes for a very high-intensity workout. With varied and unusual exercises, it is a great workout to break through boredom and physical plateaus to bring your participants' fitness to a new level. The movements are integrated with full-body focus to provide a high caloric expenditure. With different timing options, you can also build progressions within the program simply by changing the work-to-rest ratios.

SETUP AND GUIDELINES

Equipment stations are established around the training area. There are two rounds with different exercises in each, using the same equipment. A simple structure of a 1 minute of work and 15 to 30 seconds of transition time is acceptable to start. You can also add progressions by getting creative with timing, using a 20:10 work-to-rest ratio, repeated two to four times depending on the overall length of your class. You might also do just one round repeated for four sets if your class is on the shorter side.

DURATION

45 to 60 minutes

EQUIPMENT

Battle ropes, agility ladder, BOSU Balance Trainer, rowing machine, slam ball or SandBell, kettlebell

ADDITIONAL WORKOUT NOTES

- Allow 7 to 10 minutes of dynamic total-body movements to prepare for the workout. You might try using the Sample Total-Body Dynamic Warm-Up outlined in chapter 11.
- Ensure participants stay hydrated and keep the room temperature cool. HIIT workouts significantly elevate body temperature, so if you're working in a smaller space, make sure the air is circulating well and that your group has access to water. Stopping for water breaks is a very good idea.
- Because they will be sharing equipment, each person should have a towel for sweat. A BOSU Balance Trainer can be slippery when wet, so at the very least, supply a towel for this station.
- When all rounds have been completed, spend at least 7 to 10 minutes cooling down using the Sample Floor-Based Static Stretch Cool-Down from chapter 11.

Round 1	
Exercise	**Adaptations**
Row	To regress, perform 26-30 strokes per minute. To progress, perform 30-40 strokes per minute.
Battle ropes: Double-arm slams with squats (Page 197)	To regress, decrease ROM. To progress, add a jump to squat.
Agility ladder: High-speed single- and double-foot contact runs (Page 198)	To regress, decrease speed of movement. To progress, add high-knee running.
BOSU Balance Trainer: Dome squat jump (Page 198)	To regress, start jump on floor and step back down. To progress, perform a tuck jump.
Slam ball: Double-arm slams (Page 199)	To regress, decrease ROM, load, and speed. To progress, increase ROM, load, and speed.
Kettlebell: Double-arm swings (Page 199)	To regress, decrease ROM and load. To progress, increase ROM, load, and speed.
Round 2	
Exercise	**Adaptations**
Row	To regress, perform 26-30 strokes per minute. To progress, perform 30-40 strokes per minute.
Battle ropes: Alternating waves with jump lunge (Page 200)	To regress, keep it low impact and don't jump. To progress, increase speed and ROM.
Agility ladder: High-speed out-out-in-in or lateral run-throughs (Page 201)	To regress, slow down and keep knees lower. To progress, add high-knee running.
BOSU Balance Trainer: Burpee push-ups with platform side up (Page 202)	To regress, place knees on floor for push-up and walk feet in and out of plank. To progress, pick BOSU up and raise overhead.
Slam ball: Side-to-side slams	To regress, decrease load and speed. To progress, increase load and speed, and add a squat jump with each slam.
Kettlebell: Alternating single-arm swings (Page 202)	To regress, decrease load or perform double-arm swing. To progress, increase load, speed, and ROM.

Metabolic Magic Workout

This MET program focuses on integrated total-body exercises and drills, using a large amount of muscle to provide a metabolic effect. Additionally, with a high demand on the cardiovascular system provided by the battle rope drills, rowing (or running), and kettlebell exercises, the workout is designed to amplify caloric expenditure to boost fat loss. This program also provides maximum variety while still allowing for skill development—for instance, rowing is novel for many clients, but because it is repeated throughout the workout, it gives participants a chance to master the technique. For this reason, Metabolic Magic is ideal for fit, experienced participants who love a challenge and want to gain whole-body strength and cardiovascular fitness.

SETUP AND GUIDELINES

This workout comprises a total of three unique series of four different movements. The group moves through each series of four exercises with a prescribed number of repetitions, trying to complete as many rounds as possible (AMRAP) for three minutes. The individual on the rowing machine, treadmill, or bike works at hard intensity for two minutes and finishes with one minute at an anaerobic intensity. If the individual is using a treadmill, then increasing the incline rather than speed is an excellent way to create the anaerobic challenge. Allow for 45 to 60 seconds of recovery between exercises and at least one to two minutes of recovery between each series.

DURATION

45 to 60 minutes

NUMBER OF PARTICIPANTS

4

EQUIPMENT

Battle ropes, kettlebells, BOSU Balance Trainer, rowing machine (or bike or treadmill), suspension system

ADDITIONAL WORKOUT NOTES

- Allow 7 to 10 minutes of dynamic total-body movements to prepare for the workout. You might try using the Sample Total-Body Dynamic Warm-up outlined in chapter 11.
- Focus on technique and form for all exercises, especially the ropes and rowers. Both of these pieces of equipment can place stress on the lower back when performed poorly. Ensure that the spine remains neutral for the ropes and that there's full-body action with coordination among the legs, core, and upper extremities.
- This workout is extremely intense, so watch your participants carefully for any signs of overexertion, such as excessive sweating, facial redness, or breathlessness.
- Spend at least 7 to 10 minutes cooling down using the Sample Floor-Based Static Stretch Cool-Down outlined in chapter 11.

Series 1		
Exercises	**Reps/time**	**Adaptations**
Battle ropes: Double-arm slams with squats (Page 197)	10 reps	To regress, slow the movement and decrease ROM. To progress, add a squat jump.
Kettlebells: Alternating single-arm swings (Page 202)	15 reps	To regress, try a lighter load. To progress, try a heavier load.
BOSU Balance Trainer: Burpee push-ups with platform side up (Page 202)	10 reps	To regress, walk rather than jump to the plank and back. To progress, pick up the BOSU Balance Trainer overhead upon standing.
Row	28 strokes per minute for 2 minutes, then 30-40 strokes per minute for 1 minute	To regress, start at 26 strokes per minute. To progress, move to 28 strokes per minute.

Series 2		
Exercises	**Reps/time**	**Adaptations**
Battle ropes: Alternating waves (Page 203)	10 reps	To regress, slow the movement and decrease ROM. To progress, increase speed and ROM.
Kettlebell: Deadlift	10 reps	To regress, increase knee flexion and decrease load. To progress, increase load.
Suspension: Inverted rows (Page 203)	10 reps	To regress, walk feet further away from anchor point. To progress, walk feet further forward.
Row	28 strokes per minute for 2 minutes, then 30-40 strokes per minute for 1 minute	To regress, start at 26 strokes per minute. To progress, move to 28 strokes per minute.

Series 3		
Exercises	**Reps/time**	**Adaptations**
Battle ropes: Grappler throws (Page 204)	10 reps	To regress, slow the movement and decrease ROM. To progress, increase speed and ROM.
Dumbbells or kettlebells: Alternating lateral lunges	10 reps	To regress, decrease load and ROM. To progress, increase load and ROM.
Suspension: Power pull-up (Page 205)	7 reps each side	To regress, perform bilaterally. To progress, walk feet further forward.
Row	28 strokes per minute for 2 minutes, then 30-40 strokes per minute for 1 minute	To regress, start at 26 strokes per minute. To progress, move to 28 strokes per minute.

Superset Ladder Workout

This MET workout will push your participants to a new level of fitness using only dumbbells. By using simple exercises combined with an interesting repetition ladder, it will challenge muscular strength and endurance while enhancing the circulatory system through peripheral heart action. With no rest between exercises or sets, the intensity of this workout builds!

SETUP AND GUIDELINES

The repetition ladder is easy to employ. There are four sets for each superset: the first set of the superset is 8 reps, the second is 7, the third is 6, and the fourth set is 5. Participants can count their own reps. For the unilateral exercises, do each side for the prescribed repetitions, then perform the second exercise in the superset for the same reps. Complete all four sets before moving to the next superset. When all four supersets are finished, recover for 60 seconds to hydrate and towel off sweat. After all the supersets have been completed, finish the workout with the descending core ladder, following the same idea using the reps and time outlined in the program. This combination of the plank with the bicycle is intense, even though the plank is held for only 16 seconds at the longest. When combined nonstop with the bicycle, fatigue builds quickly.

To modify the workout, allow participants to rest between sets or decrease reps. You might try a progression of reps such as 5-4-3-2 to give 15 reps; any repetition range between 8 to 5 and 5 to 2 allows for progression and regression.

DURATION

45 to 60 minutes

NUMBER OF PARTICIPANTS

2 to 4

EQUIPMENT

Two dumbbells per person, one mat per person

ADDITIONAL WORKOUT NOTES

- Allow 7 to 10 minutes of dynamic total-body movements to prepare for the workout. You might try the Sample Total-Body Dynamic Warm-Up outlined in chapter 11.
- Start your participants with a lower rep range for the first sets and build as a slow progression to promote proper adaptation. As your class advances, heavier dumbbells, less rest between exercises, faster tempo, and more reps can all increase the challenge.
- Carefully observe your participants for any signs of excessive fatigue that may cause a loss of body control or coordination in order to prevent any injuries.
- Spend at least 7 to 10 minutes cooling down using the Sample Floor-Based Static Stretch Cool-Down from chapter 11.

Exercise	Sets/reps	Adaptations
1a. Two-dumbbell front and reverse lunge (Page 206) 1b. One-dumbbell diagonal chop and shoulder press (Page 207)	4 × descending reps for each superset as follows: Set 1: 8 reps each side Set 2: 7 reps each side Set 3: 6 reps each side Set 4: 5 reps each side	To regress, decrease load, tempo, or volume. To progress, increase load, tempo, or volume.
2a. Two-dumbbell single-leg deadlift and side lunge (Page 208) 2b. Two-dumbbell squat and curl (Page 209)		To regress, decrease load, tempo, or volume and keep lag foot in contact with the floor for the deadlift. To progress, increase load, tempo, or volume and lift lag leg for the deadlift.
3a. Two-dumbbell crossover lunge and side lunge (Page 210) 3b. Two-dumbbell bent-over row with deadlift (Page 211)		To regress, decrease load, tempo, or volume. For the lunges, keep ROM smaller. To progress, increase load, tempo, or volume.
4a. Two-dumbbell loaded bridge 4b. Two-dumbbell bridge with triceps extension (Page 212)		To regress, decrease load, tempo, or volume. To progress, increase load, tempo, or volume.

Exercise		Reps/time	Adaptations
Descending core ladder (4 rounds)	Slow bicycle	4 × descending reps as follows: Set 1: 8 reps Set 2: 7 reps Set 3: 6 reps Set 4: 5 reps	To regress, decrease reps or time. Recovery between exercises can also be added.
	Plank	4 × descending time as follows: Set 1: 16 s Set 2: 14 s Set 3: 12 s Set 4: 10 s	

Lean Mean Machine Workout

This calorie-torching MET workout will not only improve body composition, but also overall fitness with its metabolic effects. This workout is broken into five phases: a built-in warm-up, a conditioning phase, a core finisher, a metabolic finisher, and then a cool-down. The conditioning phase is extremely high intensity; load and speed of movement dramatically influence the intensity and cardio sprints, and significantly elevate heart rate. It is performed round-robin style, which allows participants to move within their own fitness level. This workout utilizes the AMRAP (as many rounds as possible) format, so you only need to time the overall phases; there is no need to time any of the individual exercises. This frees you up to coach and supervise closely.

SETUP AND GUIDELINES

The five phases are broken down as follows:

1. *Built-in warm-up:* 5-minute AMRAP (each round is 10 reps of 4 exercises)
2. *Conditioning phase:* 30-minute AMRAP supersets with cardio burst (12 reps of 2 exercises, then a 20-second cardio sprint); the goal is to achieve 4 rounds, but if the participant is less fit, they can do fewer
3. *Core finisher:* 3 exercises for 60 seconds each, no rest between
4. *Metabolic finisher:* 3 squat challenges for 60 seconds each, no rest between
5. *Total-body cool-down:* 5- to 10-minute cool-down using the Sample Floor-Based Static Stretch Cool-Down from chapter 11

DURATION

50 to 60 minutes

NUMBER OF PARTICIPANTS

2 to 8

EQUIPMENT

Dumbbells, kettlebells, weight bench or stability ball, rower or treadmill

ADDITIONAL WORKOUT NOTES

- Because there's such a wide variety of equipment involved in this workout, prepare the room ahead of time to ensure you have the right amount of equipment and load options available.
- Watch for any fatigue that may decrease movement precision and degrade technique. Due to the high intensity and volume of the movements, your participants my experience increased levels of fatigue.
- Make sure participants don't leave the treadmill running between sprints.
- Ensure participants stay hydrated and keep the room temperature cool. MET workouts significantly elevate body temperature, so if you're work-

ing in a smaller space, make sure the air is circulating well and that your group has access to water. Stopping for water breaks is a very good idea.

- Background music can really help motivate your group. This should not be music that you would move to on the beat, but something upbeat and appropriate to your group's taste. Because everyone is moving separately, music can add a motivating and cohesive element to your class.

Warm-up (5-min AMRAP)	Exercise	Reps	Adaptations
	Reverse lunge to overhead press (Page 213)	10 reps each	To regress, decrease load or speed of movement. Push-ups can also be done on the knees if necessary. To progress, increase load or speed of movement.
	Alt side lunge		
	Push-ups to dynamic beast (Page 213)		
	Walking plank (Page 224)		
Conditioning (30-min AMRAP)	**Exercise**	**Reps/time**	**Adaptations**
	1a. Dumbbell deadlift	12 reps each	To regress, decrease ROM and load. To progress, increase ROM and load.
	1b. Dumbbell biceps curl		
	Cardio burst on treadmill or row machine	20 s	
	2a. Kettlebell swing	12 reps each	
	2b. Kettlebell clean and press (Page 214)		
	Cardio burst on treadmill or row machine	20 s	
	3a. Dumbbell chest press	12 reps each	
	3b. Dumbbell supine triceps press		
	Cardio burst on treadmill or row machine	20 s	
	4a. Kettlebell goblet squat (Page 215)	12 reps each	
	4b. Kettlebell push press (Page 216)		
	Cardio burst on treadmill or row machine	20 s	
Core finisher (3 min)	**Exercise**	**Time**	**Adaptations**
	Mountain climber (Page 217)	1 min each	To regress, add 15-20 seconds of recovery.
	Super slow mountain climber		
	Plank		
Metabolic finisher (3 min)	**Exercise**	**Time**	**Adaptations**
	Squat jump	1 min each	To regress, decrease time and add recovery.
	Squat		
	Squat with isometric hold		
Cool-down (5-10 min)	Sample Floor-Based Static Stretch Cool-Down (chapter 11) (Page 141)		Foam rolling can be included as the stretch component.

Bigger Better Stronger Workout

This high-intensity MET workout, intended to build muscle mass and improve strength, is broken into five phases: a built-in warm-up, a strength phase, a hypertrophy phase, a metabolic finisher, and then a cool-down. The loads are heavier with fewer repetitions and include 3 to 5 sets, depending on the phase of the class. With repeat sets, participants will get a reasonably high volume of work that will help develop hypertrophy. This is a great workout for your SGT class that wants to improve upper-body muscular shape and size.

SETUP AND GUIDELINES

The five phases are as follows:

1. *Built-in warm-up:* The workout begins with a 5-minute AMRAP (10 repetitions of 5 exercises with kettlebell). This allows participants to self-regulate, because they can move at their own speed and choose the appropriate load. This specific warm-up also includes some simple bodyweight movements to integrate the core and upper body.

2. *Strength phase:* In the 20-minute strength phase, participants perform 4 to 5 sets of 4 heavy compound lift exercises for 5 repetitions each. These are performed round-robin style, with only a minute or so of recovery between exercises. The flexibility of the set design again allows participants to self-select workout intensity.

3. *Hypertrophy phase:* The 15-minute hypertrophy round comprises 6 exercises in 3 sets of 10, again performed round robin, with little rest between exercises.

4. *Metabolic finisher:* The metabolic finisher includes 5 different explosive exercises, executed for time or repetition. Allow 1 minute of recovery between each exercise. These are performed together as a group, with each person moving from exercise to exercise circuit style.

5. *Total-body cool-down:* Spend at least 5 to 10 minutes cooling down using the Sample Floor-Based Static Stretch Cool-Down from chapter 11. Foam rolling is also an excellent option to substitute stretching if you prefer.

DURATION

50 to 60 minutes

NUMBER OF PARTICIPANTS

6 to 10

EQUIPMENT

Kettlebells, dumbbells, barbells, chin-up bar, super bands, adjustable weight bench, step platform, suspension training system, medicine balls, sled and space for 25-meter sprints (or treadmill), rower

ADDITIONAL WORKOUT NOTES

This workout is equipment heavy and requires a lot of space, so the room should be carefully set up ahead of time so that you can be organized with your space and equipment.

The intensity is high, so encourage people to work at their own pace, using weights they can control with good technique. Supervise closely; the loads on this workout are heavier. The fact that the exercises in the heavy compound lifts and hypertrophy round are performed AMRAP in round-robin format will allow participants to pace themselves.

Only have the equipment out and ready for each of the phases. Put equipment away between phases where appropriate. Setting up and breaking down equipment for the different phases of the class allows for some built-in recovery time for your participants.

Ensure participants stay hydrated and keep the room temperature cool. HIIT workouts significantly elevate body temperature, so make sure the air is circulating well and that your group has access to water. Allowing water breaks between phases is a very good idea.

Background music can really help motivate your group. Because everyone is working at their own pace, upbeat music can help keep your group connected.

Keep clutter out of the space, especially for the metabolic finisher.

Warm-up (5-min AMRAP)	Exercise	Reps	Adaptations
	Goblet squat	10 reps each	Keep kettlebells relatively light and allow participants to work at their own speed.
	Kettlebell light swing		
	Bilateral push press		
	Walking push-up		
	Spiderman plank (Page 218)		
Strength (20 min)	**Exercise**	**Sets/reps**	**Adaptations**
	Kettlebell heavy deadlift	5 reps × 4-5 sets	Choose loads that fatigue the muscles in the prescribed rep ranges. The super band allows participants the opportunity to progress to bodyweight chin-ups.
	Dumbbell chest press		
	Dumbbell squat and press		
	Super band pull-up (Page 218)		
Hypertrophy (15 min)	**Exercise**	**Sets/reps**	**Adaptations**
	Barbell bent-over row	10 reps × 3 sets (each side when applicable)	Choose loads that fatigue the muscles in the prescribed rep ranges and take only as much rest as needed.
	Kettlebell single-arm bent-over row		
	Dumbbell incline chest press		
	Dumbbell single-arm incline chest press		
	Suspension supine hamstring curl (Page 219)		
	Platform lateral step-up		
Metabolic finisher	**Exercise**	**Time/reps**	**Adaptations**
	Sled push (Page 220)	1 min	
	Rowing sprint	1 min	
	Push-up	50 reps	
	25-meter sprint	5 sprints	
	Medicine ball Russian twist (Page 221)	50 reps	
Cool-down (5-10 min)	Sample Floor-Based Static Stretch Cool-Down (Page 141) (see chapter 11)		Foam rolling can be included as the stretch component.

Lose That Last 10 Workout

Anyone who's on a weight loss journey, whether they've lost a lot or a little, knows that last 10 pounds is always the hardest! More than anything, weight loss depends on optimal eating habits, but having the right calorie-torching program can help make that final 10 easier to lose. Having fun while doing it? That just makes it something to look forward to.

This HIIT cardio workout uses timed drills with the whole group working together, making it easy to coach. The movements are simple, functional, and athletic. The BOSU Balance Trainer creates a whole new level of challenge that increases intensity, complexity, and coordination demands. HIIT cardio on the BOSU Balance Trainer drives heart rate up, enhancing cardiovascular fitness, caloric expenditure, and EPOC.

SETUP AND GUIDELINES

Typically, this is a 60-minute workout, with each movement series performed for a total of 3 minutes (1 minute per exercise) and a recovery period of 60 seconds before moving to the next series. However, length can be adjusted depending on your time, so if you only have 30 minutes, you could perform each series for 90 seconds (30 seconds per exercise), then recover for 30 seconds.

Each exercise progresses a series of movements through speed and ROM. The first minute is spent moving slower, focusing on control, balance, and posture. The second minute increases tempo and the third minute is performed explosively. This triplet sequence builds motor learning—the first movement teaches the second movement and the second teaches the third. This invisible teaching allows participants to learn the movements thoroughly before they move explosively. It also builds in a regression, providing a multilevel teaching option. For a less-conditioned participant, they have the option to omit the explosive movement and simply do the second exercise for longer.

As the coach, you can also omit the third movement entirely or decrease the time. For example, perform the first two drills for 45 seconds and the third for 30. This shortens the workout, decreases the intensity and volume, and allows participants to progress gradually. For stronger, fitter groups, doing the full minute of each drill will create an intense cardiovascular challenge!

EQUIPMENT

BOSU Balance Trainer

DURATION

60 minutes (can be adjusted as needed)

ADDITIONAL WORKOUT NOTES

- Participants should wear shoes with good lateral support; running shoes are not recommended. A cross-training shoe that's flat and laced firmly is the best option.
- The Balance Trainer is extremely slippery when wet, so a towel should be kept handy to wipe off sweat.

- Ensure participants stay hydrated and keep the room temperature cool. HIIT workouts significantly elevate body temperature, so if you're working in a smaller space, make sure the air is circulating well and that your group has access to water. Allowing water breaks between each series is a very good idea.

- Whether you choose to move to the beat or simply have it in the background, this high-intensity workout runs well with music. Rhythmic workouts operate well when people are moving in unison, so it can make sense to use the beat to motivate your group. One of the advantages of not moving rhythmically, however, is that it allows people to move at their own speed, with their own sense of rhythm and timing, which is especially critical when working with an unstable surface like a BOSU Balance Trainer. This can be especially helpful for groups with mixed skill level. Having music in the background can accommodate these differences.

- Spend at least 7 to 10 minutes cooling down using the Sample Floor-Based Static Stretch Cool-Down from chapter 11.

Warm-up (6-7 min)	Exercise	Time	Adaptations
	Squat on top of BOSU Balance Trainer	1 min	To regress, slow the movements (but still perform each movement for 1 minute). To progress, increase speed and ROM.
	March/jog/run (dome side)	1-2 min	
	Walking burpee (dome side)	1 min	
	Alternating dome lunge (dome side) (Page 222)	1 min	
	Walking push-up (dome side)	1 min	

Series 1 (3 min)			
Exercise		Time	Adaptations
Side-to-side squat (slow; dome side)		1 min each	To regress, decrease speed, ROM, or time.
Side-to-side squat jump and stick on top of BOSU Balance Trainer (faster; dome side) (Page 223)			
Side-to-side squat jump (fast; dome side)			

Series 2 (3 min)			
Exercise		Time	Adaptations
Walking plank (slow; dome side)		1 min each	To regress, decrease speed, ROM, or time.
Jump to plank then perform two plank jacks (faster; dome side)			
Burpee plank jacks (fast; dome side)			

Series 3 (3 min)			
Exercise		Reps/time	Adaptations
Rear lunge knee touch on top of BOSU Balance Trainer (slow) (Page 225)		4 × 1 min each side	To regress, decrease speed, ROM, or time.
Rear lunge knee touch on top of BOSU Balance Trainer (faster) (Page 225)		2 × 1 min each side	
Rear lunge jump on top of BOSU Balance Trainer (fast)		Alternate sides for 1 min	

(continued)

Lose That Last 10 Workout *(continued)*

Series 4 (3 min)		
Exercise	**Time**	**Adaptations**
Straddle down to dome plank with hands on dome, then perform 4 alternating lunges (slow) (Page 222)	1 min each	To regress, decrease speed, ROM, or time.
Straddle down to dome plank with hands on dome, then perform 4 alternating jump lunges (faster)		
Jump and straddle down to dome plank with hands on dome, then perform 4 alternating jump lunges (fast)		
Series 5 (3 min)		
Exercise	**Time**	**Adaptations**
Stand to the right of BOSU Balance Trainer, step up and down on the right side one time, then over to the other side, stepping up and down one time, then repeat (slow)	1 min each	To regress, decrease speed, ROM, or time.
Stand to the right of BOSU Balance Trainer, step up and down on the right side one time, then over to the other side, stepping up and down one time, then repeat (faster)		
Stand to the right of BOSU Balance Trainer, step up and down on the right side one time, then jump over to the other side, stepping up and down one time, then repeat (fast)		
Series 6 (3 min)		
Exercise	**Time**	**Adaptations**
Step up and balance on right leg, step down, repeat step up and balance on left leg, then walk down to plank (slow)	1 min each	To regress, decrease speed, ROM, or time.
Jump up and balance on right leg, step down, repeat jump up and balance on left leg, then walk down to plank (faster)		
Jump up and balance on right leg, step down, repeat jump up and balance on left leg, then perform a burpee (fast)		
Series 7 (3 min)		
Exercise	**Time**	**Adaptations**
Straddle down and up (slow)	1 min each	To regress, decrease speed, ROM, or time.
Straddle down and jump up (faster)		
Jump and straddle down and up (fast)		

Partner and Team Training Programs

One of the main advantages of partner and team training in a small-group setting is that it provides an excellent opportunity to build community and accountability in a more social environment. Participants develop bonds and become accountable to each other as well as to the group as a whole. This helps build consistency in attendance and makes it easier for you to retain clients. It can also provide some healthy competition and will help build camaraderie.

Partner training is also an ideal way to cut down on equipment needs. If you have a larger group of six or more, then circuit training is the perfect solution. Note, however, that when guiding participants in this setting, instruction needs to be clear and concise! When your group is talking, laughing, and working together, it is easy for the class to become out of control, so your cueing needs to be simple and easy to understand.

Partner Play Workout

This partner workout is designed to enhance muscular strength and endurance while simultaneously improving functional whole-body integration. The exercises all rely on a coordinated effort between partners. Participants not only have to move efficiently as individuals, but must also synchronize timing and rhythm with their partner.

SETUP AND GUIDELINES

This program has four series; each full series is performed twice in order, with 60 seconds of recovery between each series. Each exercise should be performed for 60 seconds with 15 to 20 seconds of transition and rest between exercises.

DURATION

45 minutes

NUMBER OF PARTICIPANTS

4 to 6 (2-3 partners)

EQUIPMENT

Resistance bands

ADDITIONAL WORKOUT NOTES

- Allow 5 to 7 minutes of dynamic total-body movements to prepare for the workout. You might try the Sample Total-Body Dynamic Warm-Up outlined in chapter 11.
- Try to partner clients of similar size and fitness levels. Pairing similar-sized individuals optimizes the line-of-pull angle for exercises using resistance bands. Pairing fitter individuals can also provide a little more challenge through some friendly competitiveness, and they will also be more likely to work with similar levels of resistance and load, making equipment selection easier. If you have an uneven number of people, partner up with the least strong person so you can give them a little more encouragement.
- Choose the participant with the best coordination and body control to use as a partner to demonstrate each drill. This way you'll be able to provide the best possible demonstration while still accommodating less-conditioned folks.
- Regularly inspect your rubber resistance bands for wear and tear, and dispose of any worn or damaged bands.
- By nature, elastic resistance is unique compared to equipment like dumbbells or barbells. Always focus on controlling the eccentric phase of each movement to resist the elastic recoil of the band.
- At the completion of the workout, be sure to provide your class with plenty of time to cool down. This is a great opportunity to improve flexibility and develop good stretching habits (see Sample Floor-Based Static Stretch Cool-Down, chapter 11).

Series 1		
Exercise	**Sets/time**	**Adaptations**
Split squat and bow-and-arrow pull (1 resistance band per pair) (Page 226)	2 × 1 min each with 15-20 s rest between exercises. Allow 60 s recovery between each series.	To progress, try a heavier resistance band or stand with feet further apart. To regress, leave knees on the floor. To progress, lift top foot into a star position.
Transverse lunge with sword draw (1 resistance band per pair) (Page 234)		
Side plank and row (1 resistance band per pair) (Page 227)		

Series 2		
Exercise	**Sets/time**	**Adaptations**
Squat and high pull (1 resistance band per person) (Page 228)	2 × 1 min each with 15-20 s rest between exercises. Allow 60 s recovery between each series.	To progress, try a heavier resistance band or stand with feet further apart.
Front lunge and chop (1 resistance band per pair) (Page 228)		
Side-by-side front chop (1 resistance band per pair)		

Series 3		
Exercise	**Sets/time**	**Adaptations**
Chain-gang squat (1 resistance band per pair) (Page 229)	2 × 1 min each with 15-20 s rest between exercises. Allow 60 s recovery between series.	To progress, try a heavier resistance band or stand with feet further apart.
Chest press with front lunge (1 resistance band per person) (Page 230)		
Side-by-side alternating chop (1 resistance band per pair) (Page 231)		

Series 4		
Exercise	**Sets/time**	**Adaptations**
Side lunge with high pull (1 resistance band per pair) (Page 232)	2 × 1 min each with 15-20 s rest between series	To progress, try a heavier resistance band or stand with feet further apart.
Push-up with high-five		To regress, leave knees on ground. To progress, lift opposite foot from the floor with the high-five.
Partner bicycle (Page 233)		To regress, place a small ball behind lower back to add support. To progress, sit taller and lift hands from the floor.

Circuit Solutions Workout

This circuit training workout is simple to teach and fun and effective for your participants. It uses naturally integrated, functional, and core-centric suspension training combined with dumbbell and resistance tube exercises to create a well-balanced workout. Although most of the exercises are performed solo, there are a few partner drills. This builds camaraderie and socialization, generating a team feel throughout the workout.

SETUP AND GUIDELINES

This workout is structured as a mini-circuit with timed stations. There are a total of three stations with four exercises in each. Perform 2 to 3 sets of 45 to 60 seconds per exercise before moving to the next series. Use 10 to 15 seconds of transition between exercises and 30 to 60 seconds of recovery between series.

DURATION

45 to 60 minutes

NUMBER OF PARTICIPANTS

4 to 8

EQUIPMENT

Suspension training system, dumbbells, step platform, resistance bands

ADDITIONAL WORKOUT NOTES

- Allow 5 to 7 minutes of dynamic total-body movements to prepare for the workout. You might try the Sample Total-Body Dynamic Warm-Up as outlined in chapter 11.
- Try to partner clients of similar size and fitness levels. Pairing similar-sized individuals optimizes the line-of-pull angle for exercises using resistance bands. Pairing those with similar strength levels also allows them to share the equipment, wherever possible.
- For less-conditioned individuals, decrease work time and increase recovery times. Once people are familiar with the workout, you can increase the challenge by shortening recovery times.
- The first time you introduce this workout to your group, you may only have time for two sets. As they familiarize, add in the third set, if time permits.
- At the completion of the workout, be sure to provide your class with plenty of time to cool down. This is a great opportunity to improve flexibility and develop good stretching habits (see Sample Floor-Based Static Stretch Cool-Down, chapter 11).

Series 1		
Exercise	**Sets/time**	**Adaptations**
Suspension chest press	2-3 × 45-60 s each with 10-15 s rest between exercises. Allow 30-60 s recovery between sets	To regress, start in a more upright position. To progress, move into a more inclined position.
Kettlebell goblet squat (Page 215)		To progress, deepen ROM and choose a heavier load.
Resistance bands partner split squat and row (Page 234)		To progress, try a heavier resistance band or stand with feet further apart.
Kettlebell push press (Page 216)		To regress, try alternating presses, or use a lighter load. To progress, try a heavier load.

Series 2		
Exercise	**Sets/time**	**Adaptations**
Suspension pull	2-3 × 45-60 s each with 10-15 s rest between exercises. Allow 30-60 s recovery between sets.	To regress, start in a more upright position. To progress, start at a greater reclining angle and lift one foot off the floor.
Dumbbell lateral step-up		To progress, try a higher step and heavier load.
Transverse lunge and sword draw (Page 234)		To progress, try a heavier resistance band or stand with feet further apart.
Dumbbell squat curl and press (Page 192)		To progress, increase ROM and try a heavier load.

Series 3		
Exercise	**Sets/time**	**Adaptations**
Suspension single-leg squat and row (Page 230)	2-3 × 45-60 s each with 10-15 s rest between exercises. Allow 30-60 s recovery between sets.	To regress, start in a more upright position or perform a bilateral squat. To progress, start at a greater incline.
Dumbbell deadlift		To regress, decrease ROM and load. To progress, increase ROM and load.
Front lunge and chop (Page 228)		To progress, try a heavier resistance band or stand with feet further apart.
Dumbbell supine bridge and pull-over (Page 195)		To progress, place feet on the platform side of a BOSU Balance Trainer.

Double Trouble Workout

The Double Trouble Workout takes it up a notch by adding some explosive movement using kettlebells and medicine balls. This partner training program is a progression in intensity from the previous two workouts, so make sure your group is ready for it. Although it's a fully scalable workout, the kettlebell exercises require learned skills such as deadlifting and squatting and use ballistic-type action along with overhead movements that require high levels of shoulder stability and strength. Partner Play is a better introductory program, so save this one for further down the line.

SETUP AND GUIDELINES

This workout uses compound, integrated exercises that focus on total-body function to not only enhance muscular strength and endurance, but also improve hand–eye coordination, balance, core mobility, and stability. It also includes a fun built-in ladder warm-up of simple, familiar exercises using a medicine ball and bodyweight movements. Perform 1 to 2 sets of each series before moving to the next, doing 45 to 60 seconds per exercise. Use 10 to 15 seconds of transition and rest between exercises and 20 to 30 seconds of recovery between series.

DURATION

45 to 60 minutes

NUMBER OF PARTICIPANTS

2 to 8

EQUIPMENT

Kettlebell, medicine ball (one per pair)

ADDITIONAL WORKOUT NOTES

- The load of kettlebells and medicine balls needs to be appropriate for the strength and fitness levels of your participants. Additionally, it's a good idea to make sure your group can squat and deadlift with correct technique before performing ballistic kettlebell exercises.
- To create a team environment, pair clients of similar strength and have them switch off between equipment and exercises. If performing two sets of each exercise, for example, partner A does the kettlebell movement while the partner B does the medicine ball drill for the prescribed time; then they switch. This is then repeated for a second set. Have them face each other while working and encourage them to coach and cheer. For a competitive challenge, have them count their reps and keep a tally on a leaderboard. At the end of the workout, the partners with the highest reps win a prize!
- At the completion of the workout, be sure to provide your class with plenty of time to cool down. This is a great opportunity to improve flexibility and develop good stretching habits (see Sample Floor-Based Static Stretch Cool-Down, chapter 11).

Partner warm-up		
Exercise	**Reps**	**Adaptations**
Squat	At a steady tempo, perform 5 reps of each circuit with no rest between exercises. Follow this with a circuit of 4 reps each, then 3, 2, and 1, for a total of 15 reps.	To regress, move slower and focus on technique and form, and add rest between sets. To progress, perform the entire warm-up with no rest between exercises and sets.
Push-ups to dynamic beast (Page 213)		
Reverse lunge		
Medicine ball push press		

Series 1		
Exercise	**Reps/sets/time**	**Adaptations**
Medicine ball front lunge with over-head chop and rotation (Page 236)	1-2 × 45-60 s each with 10-15 s rest between each exercise. Allow 20-30 s recovery between sets.	To regress the medicine ball exercise, hold the medicine ball at chest and avoid overhead movement. To regress the kettlebell exercise, pass the kettlebell over front thigh. To progress, choose heavier loads.
Kettlebell reverse lunge with figure-8 pass under leg		

Series 2		
Exercise	**Reps/sets/time**	**Adaptations**
Medicine ball squat swing and toss (Page 237)	1-2 × 45-60 s each with 10-15 s rest between each exercise. Allow 20-30 s recovery between sets.	To regress the medicine ball exercise, remove the toss. To regress the kettlebell exercise, perform as a goblet squat. To progress, choose heavier loads.
Kettlebell swing		

Series 3		
Exercise	**Reps/sets/time**	**Adaptations**
Medicine ball 1-2 Russian twist with curtsy lunge (Page 221)	1-2 × 45-60 s each with 10-15 s rest between each exercise. Allow 20-30 s recovery between sets.	To regress the medicine ball exercise, decrease the tempo. To regress the kettlebell exercise, leave the other toe on the floor. To progress, increase tempo and load, and raise the rear leg on the deadlift movement.
Kettlebell single-leg deadlift		

Series 4		
Exercise	**Reps/sets/time**	**Adaptations**
Medicine ball side lunge with overhead chop with rotation (Page 238)	1-2 × 45-60 s each with 10-15 s rest between each exercise. Allow 20-30 s recovery between sets.	To regress the medicine ball exercise, hold the medicine ball at the chest and omit overhead move-ment. To regress the kettlebell exercise, hold the kettlebell steady and omit the swing. To progress, increase load and tempo.
Kettlebell side lunge and swing (Page 239)		

Series 5		
Exercise	**Reps/sets/time**	**Adaptations**
Medicine ball reverse lunge with rota-tion	1-2 × 45-60 s each with 10-15 s rest between each exercise. Allow 20-30 s recovery between sets.	To regress the medicine ball exercise, keep elbows bent and med-icine ball at the chest. To regress the kettlebell exercise, perform a double-arm swing. To progress, increase load and tempo.
Kettlebell clean and press with alter-nating single-arm swing (Page 214)		

(continued)

Double Trouble Workout *(continued)*

Series 6		
Exercise	**Reps/sets/time**	**Adaptations**
Medicine ball transverse lunge with rotation (Page 240)	1-2 × 45-60 s each with 10-15 s rest between each exercise. Allow 20-30 s recovery between sets.	To regress the medicine ball exercise, decrease ROM. To regress the kettlebell exercise, omit the overhead press. To progress, increase load and tempo.
Kettlebell front lunge and overhead press (Page 240)		

Series 7		
Exercise	**Reps/sets/time**	**Adaptations**
Medicine ball overhead squat	1-2 × 45-60 s each with 10-15 s rest between each exercise. Allow 20-30 s recovery between sets.	To regress the medicine ball exercise, hold the medicine ball at chest. To regress the kettlebell exercise, hold the kettlebell with arms straight and low between the legs. To progress, add load and tempo.
Kettlebell goblet squat (Page 215)		

Series 8		
Exercise	**Reps/sets/time**	**Adaptations**
Medicine ball squat with reverse lunge and overhead press (Page 241)	1-2 × 45-60 s each with 10-15 s rest between each exercise. Allow 20-30 s recovery between sets.	To regress the medicine ball exercise, keep the medicine ball at the chest and omit the overhead press. To regress the kettlebell exercise, maintain a low windmill. To progress, add load or add impact and tempo to the medicine ball exercise.
Kettlebell windmill (Page 241)		

Series 9		
Exercise	**Reps/sets/time**	**Adaptations**
Medicine ball curtsy lunge and ball bounce (Page 242)	1-2 × 45-60 s each with 10-15 s rest between each exercise. Allow 20-30 s recovery between sets.	To regress the medicine ball exercise, slow the movement and omit the bounce. To regress the kettlebell exercise, omit the overhead press. To progress, add load or add impact and tempo to the medicine ball exercise.
Kettlebell racked front squat to reverse lunge with overhead press (Page 243)		

Series 10		
Exercise	**Reps/sets/time**	**Adaptations**
Medicine ball alternating side lunge with ball toss	1-2 × 45-60 s each with 10-15 s rest between each exercise. Allow 20-30 s recovery between sets.	To regress the medicine ball exercise, omit the toss, holding the medicine ball at chest. To regress the kettlebell exercise, perform a double-arm swing. To progress, add load or add impact and tempo to the medicine ball exercise.
Kettlebell alternating single-arm swing ladder (descending reps)		

Selected Exercises

In this final chapter you'll find descriptions of some of the exercises in chapters 12 through 14. Each exercise is broken down into its essential movements so you can easily understand the execution; however, note that it's impossible to completely describe all aspects of each movement, especially for exercises that are multifaceted, multiplanar, and dynamic. You may use each program as a template and substitute similar exercises or use modifications according to your clients' needs and equipment availability.

Dumbbell Lateral Lunge

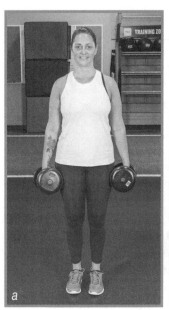
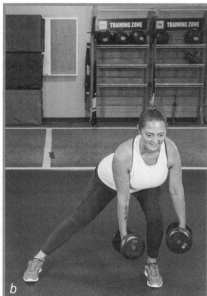

SETUP

Stand tall with the core engaged and feet together. Hold a dumbbell in each hand with arms straight at your sides (see figure *a*).

EXECUTION

Inhale and step laterally to the left, flexing the left knee, hip, and ankle while maintaining parallel alignment of the feet. Reach down to mid-shin height with dumbbells on either side of the left shin (see figure *b*). Keep the right leg extended and press hips back. Exhale and push back to the starting position. Repeat on the other side.

Resistance Band Sword Draw

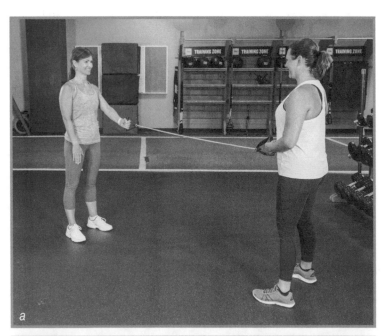

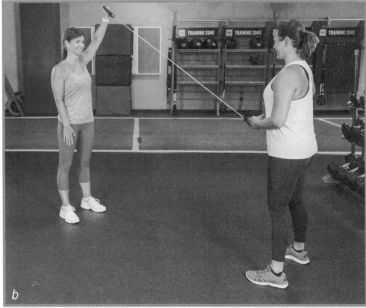

SETUP

Stand tall in a parallel stance, facing your partner (or attachment point). Hold the handle of the resistance band in the left hand (see figure *a* for an example of how the band is set up with a partner).

EXECUTION

Exhale and pull the band back diagonally in an arc while rotating the upper back and shoulder (see figure *b*). Hold for a second before inhaling and slowly returning to the starting position.

Resistance Band Triceps Walk-Back Draw

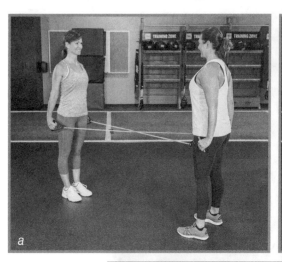
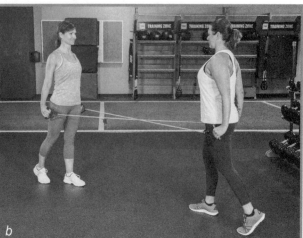

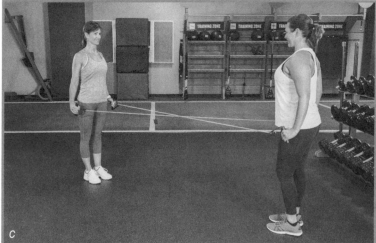

SETUP

Stand tall facing your partner (or attachment point) with arms straight down by your sides, holding the handle of a resistance band in each hand (see figure *a* for an example of how the bands are set up with a partner). Pull shoulders back and down, drawing shoulder blades together while lifting the chest.

EXECUTION

Holding hands and arms stationary, take a step backward with one foot, then the other to increase the resistance (see figures *b* and *c*). Return to the starting position in the same manner. Maintain arm and shoulder position for the whole set. Maintain a continuous breath.

Side Plank

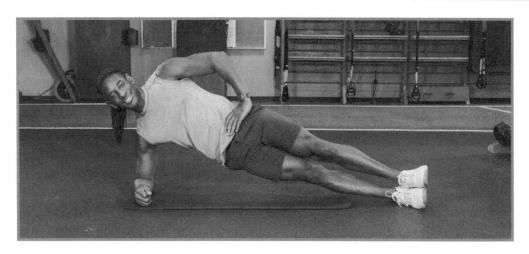

SETUP

Lie on your right side, with the right elbow directly under the shoulder, resting on forearm. Press the right shoulder down away from the ear. Place left hand on the left hip. Align legs, hips, and shoulders so the body is in a straight line.

EXECUTION

Raise hips off the floor, maintaining a long straight line from head to heels with the shoulders and hips stacked (see figure). Maintain a continuous breath.

Suspension I-Y-W-T

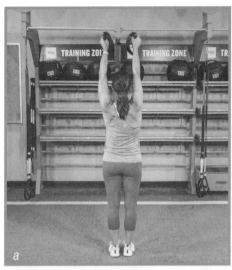

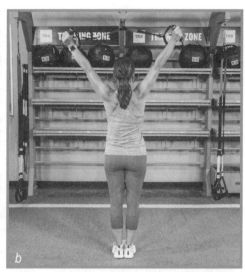

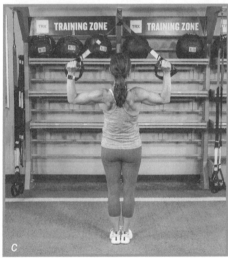

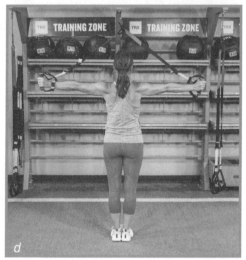

SETUP

Stand tall facing the attachment point of a suspension system. Hold the handles with arms extended and shoulders flexed to shoulder height, with the body positioned in a slight recline. There should be no slack in the suspension straps.

EXECUTION

Raise arms directly overhead, maintaining straight arms into an "I" position (see figure *a*). Return arms to the starting position. Next, raise arms diagonally upward into a "Y" position (see figure *b*). Return arms to the starting position. Now, bend the elbows and raise arms to the side into a "W" position (see figure *c*). Return arms to the starting position. Finally, horizontally abduct the arms into a "T" position, pulling shoulder blades together (see figure *d*). Keep elbows extended and return to the starting position. The body will pull forward and become more upright with each position. Keep the body rigid and stabilize through the core throughout the entire exercise. Maintain a continuous breath.

Stability Ball Hamstring Curl

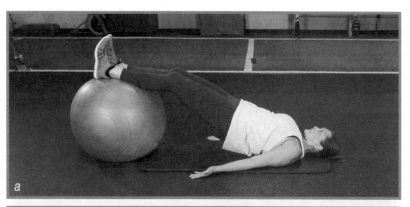

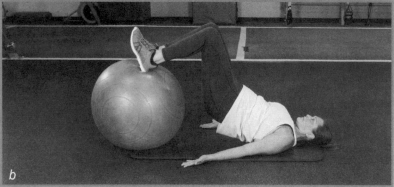

SETUP

Lie supine with feet and ankles resting on top of a stability ball and the legs extended. Turn the palms of the hands to face upwards; roll shoulders down and back.

EXECUTION

Raise hips off floor, creating a straight line from the heels to the shoulders. Keep feet parallel (see figure *a*). Bend knees and roll the ball toward the hips while maintaining hip extension (see figure *b*). Extend the knees, rolling the ball away from hips until knees are again extended, then lower the hips to the starting position. Maintain a continuous breath.

Stability Ball Plank

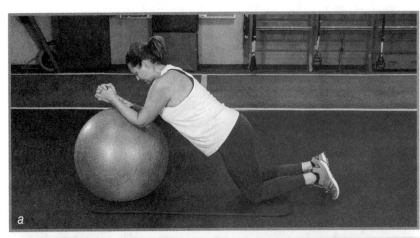

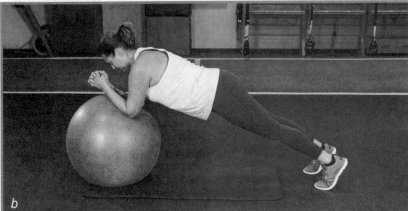

SETUP

Kneel behind a stability ball with forearms resting on top and shoulders directly over or slightly forward of the elbows (see figure *a*). Hips should be extended with a straight line from knees to shoulders.

EXECUTION

Tuck the toes under and extend the knees to hold a straight line from heels to shoulders (see figure *b*). Maintain a continuous breath.

Suspension Crossover Lunge and Pull

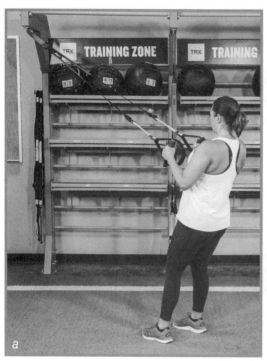 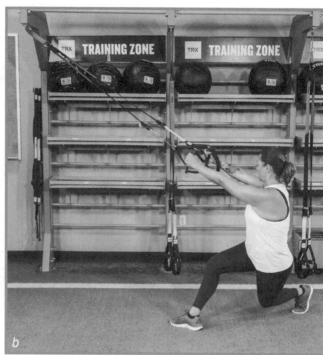

SETUP

Stand tall facing the attachment point of a suspension system. Hold the handles with elbows bent and tucked into the sides of the rib cage, with palms facing inwards. Keep a rigid body position with a slight lean back (see figure *a*).

EXECUTION

Standing on the right leg, inhale and cross the left leg behind the right leg, bending both knees while leaning back and extending the elbows (see figure *b*). At the lowered position, elbows should be fully extended and knees and hips flexed deeply with most of the body weight on the right foot. Exhale and pull the body upright to the start position. Repeat for repetitions or alternate sides.

Resistance Band Isometric Rotator Cuff Lateral Step-Out

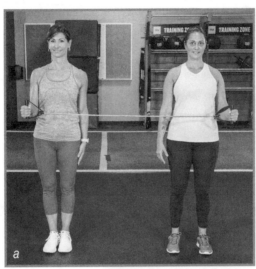
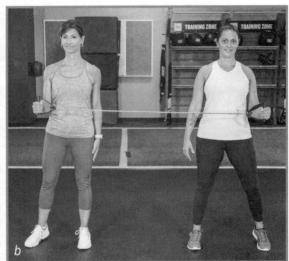
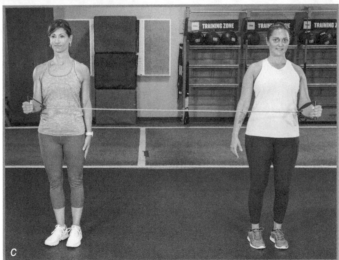

SETUP

Stand tall with feet together or slightly less than shoulder-width apart in a position side-on to a partner (or attachment point). Hold the resistance band in the hand further away from the partner or attachment point. Keep the wrist straight and the elbow bent at 90 degrees, tucked into the side of the rib cage (see figure *a*). You may want to fold a small towel and tuck it between the ribs and elbow if this position is uncomfortable.

EXECUTION

Maintaining the hand, wrist, and elbow alignment in an isometric position so there is no movement, step laterally with both feet away from the partner or attachment point (see figures *b* and *c*). Slowly step back to the starting position. Repeat this foot pattern while keeping the shoulder down and the hand, elbow, and wrist static. Maintain a continuous breath.

Resistance Band Lunge and Bow and Arrow

SETUP

In a staggered stance with the left leg forward and right leg back, flex the knees and hips to lower into a split squat. Hold the handle of a resistance band in the right hand. The left arm is at shoulder height with the elbow bent like a bow and arrow. The thoracic spine is rotated to "open" the chest.

EXECUTION

Exhale and pull the handle of the band towards the rib cage, stepping the left foot back to meet the right foot while extending the hips and knees to an upright position. Simultaneously, rotate the left hand to reach towards the band, like a bow and arrow. Inhale and return to the starting position.

Bodyweight Plank With Hip Rotation

SETUP

Assume a prone plank position, resting on the forearms with the elbows bent, the hips and knees extended, and the core braced tightly. Feet should be shoulder-width apart or slightly wider.

EXECUTION

While maintaining core strength, rotate the hips, lowering the right hip towards the floor and rotating the feet to follow. Return to the starting position and repeat on the other side. Be sure that the elbows maintain contact with the floor at all times. Maintain a continuous breath.

Dumbbell Reverse Lunge

SETUP

Stand tall with the feet together. Hold a dumbbell in each hand at your sides with the shoulders pulled back, the chest open, and the core engaged.

EXECUTION

Inhale and take a large step backward with the left foot. The ball of the left foot rests on the floor with the heel lifted. Flex the knees and hips, lowering the left knee toward the floor while the upper body remains upright. Press the right heel into the floor, exhale and return to the starting position. Repeat for repetitions or alternate sides.

POSTURE PERFECT WORKOUT

FUNCTIONAL ACTIVE AND AGING WORKOUT

Deadlift With Bent-Over Row

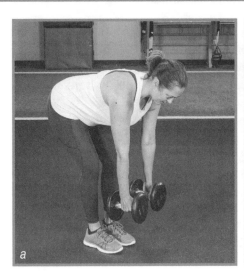 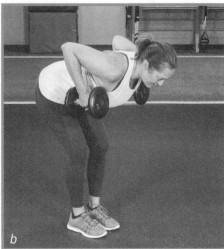

SETUP

Stand tall with the feet together. Hold a dumbbell in each hand at your sides, keeping the knees soft, shoulders down and back, and core engaged.

EXECUTION

Hinge forward at hips to approximately 90 degrees, pressing the hips back and bending knees slightly. Maintain a long, neutral spine and neck and extend the arms toward the floor (see figure *a*). Perform a row with both arms, driving the elbows toward the ceiling and pulling the shoulder blades together (see figure *b*). Lower the arms by straightening the elbows, then stand back upright to the starting position. Maintain a continuous breath.

Partner Side-By-Side Sagittal Chop

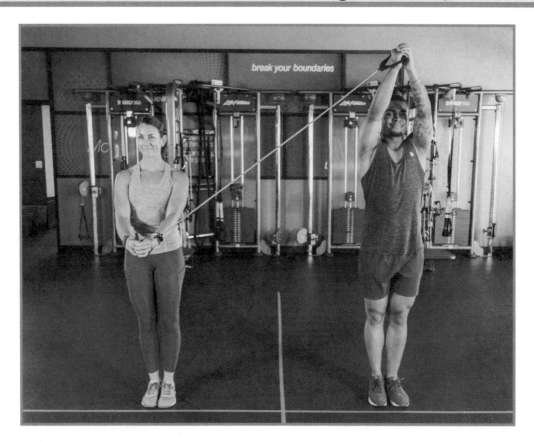

SETUP

Stand tall with feet together side-on to a partner (or attachment point). Hold a resistance band in both hands with one hand covering the other and thumbs looped around the handle. Raise the arms to shoulder height with the elbows extended, maintaining light tension on the band.

EXECUTION

Partner A lowers their hands level with the groin and partner B raises their hands directly up (in the sagittal plane) to an overhead position (see figure). Then, partner A raises their hands overhead while partner B lowers theirs level with the groin. Stay in the sagittal plane. Maintain a continuous breath.

Dumbbell Squat Curl and Press

SETUP

Stand tall with feet hip-width apart. Hold a dumbbell in each hand with the arms straight by your sides.

EXECUTION

Keeping the eyes forward, inhale and squat, lowering the dumbbells to shin level. Exhale and stand up, flexing the elbows to bring the hands to the shoulders with palms facing inwards (like a hammer curl). Inhale again, then exhale and press the dumbbells overhead, extending the elbows while keeping the palms of the hands facing inwards. Inhale and lower to the squat again as the arms lower toward the floor.

Partner Side-By-Side Alternating Rotation

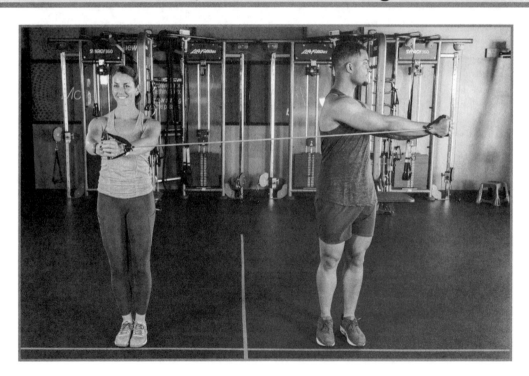

SETUP

Stand tall with feet together side-on to a partner (or attachment point). Hold a resistance band in both hands, with one hand covering the other and thumbs looped around the handle. Raise arms to shoulder height with the elbows extended, maintaining light tension on band.

EXECUTION

While partner A rotates away, partner B maintains a stable, upright position and resists the rotation (see figure). When partner A rotates back to the starting position, partner B then performs the rotation. Maintain a continuous breath.

Dumbbell or Bodyweight Transverse Lunge

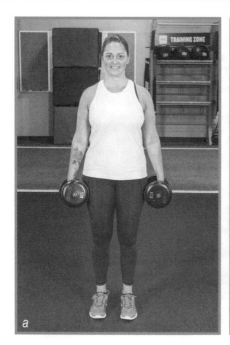
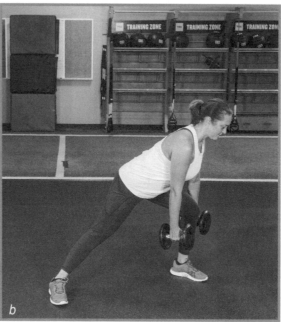

SETUP

Stand tall with the feet together. Hold a dumbbell in each hand with the arms straight at your sides (see figure *a*). Imagine you are standing on the face of a clock, with feet at 12 o'clock.

EXECUTION

Inhale and step the left leg diagonally backwards to 8 o'clock, then bend the left knee and sit the hips back. Allow the arms to lower to the left shin. Maintain the right foot at 12 o'clock (see figure *b*). Exhale and push the left leg back to the 12 o'clock position. Repeat on the right side, stepping back to 4 o'clock.

Dumbbell Step-Up With Biceps Curl

SETUP

Stand tall with the feet together behind a step platform. Hold a dumbbell in each hand at your sides. Step the right foot up onto the platform and transfer weight onto that foot.

EXECUTION

Exhale, stand all the way up onto the platform, and perform a biceps curl, flexing the elbows and bringing the hands to the shoulders. Inhale and lower back down to the floor, lowering hands to the sides. Leave the right foot on the platform and repeat for repetitions.

Dumbbell Golf Chop

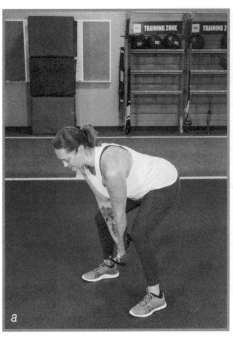 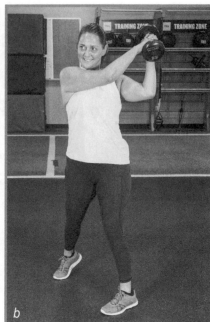

SETUP

Stand tall with feet shoulder-width apart and slightly turned out. Hold a dumbbell in both hands with fingers linked and thumbs looped around the handle. The arms are straight in a lowered position in front of the groin.

EXECUTION

Inhale and squat down, bending the knees and pressing the hips back, while swinging the dumbbell between the legs (see figure *a*). Exhale and stand explosively upright while pivoting the right foot and hip, chopping the dumbbell over the left shoulder (see figure *b*). Maintain good abdominal stability by keeping the navel pulled towards the spine. Swing the dumbbell back between the legs, pivoting the feet back to the starting position. Repeat to the other side, then keep alternating for reps or time.

Dumbbell Supine Bridge and Pullover

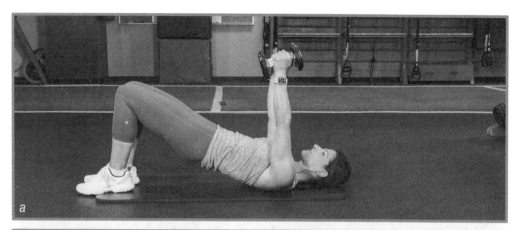

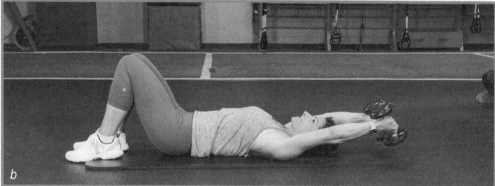

SETUP

Lie in a supine position with the knees bent and feet close to the buttocks, about hip-width apart. Hold a dumbbell directly above the chest with elbows fully extended. Raise hips into a bridge position, pointing the tailbone towards the ceiling and tucking the pelvis into a posterior pelvic tilt (see figure *a*).

EXECUTION

Inhale and simultaneously lower the hips towards the floor while lowering the dumbbell over the head, keeping the elbows extended (see figure *b*). Move in a pain-free ROM, lowering the dumbbell until the arms are close to the floor. Keep the abdominals engaged. Exhale and raise hips and arms together to return to the starting position. Repeat slowly with control.

Bird Dog

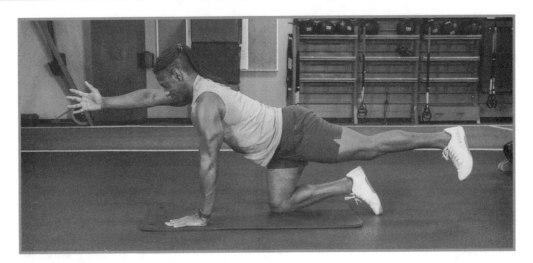

SETUP

Assume a quadruped position with the hands directly under the shoulders and knees under the hips. Find a neutral spinal position and engage the core by pulling the navel to the spine.

EXECUTION

Deeply inhale, then on an exhalation, raise the right arm and left leg until they are level with the torso (see figure). Think of stretching while maintaining a level pelvis and neutral spine. Inhale and lower before performing on the other side.

SELECTED EXERCISES FOR CHAPTER 13

Battle Ropes: Double-Arm Slams With Squats

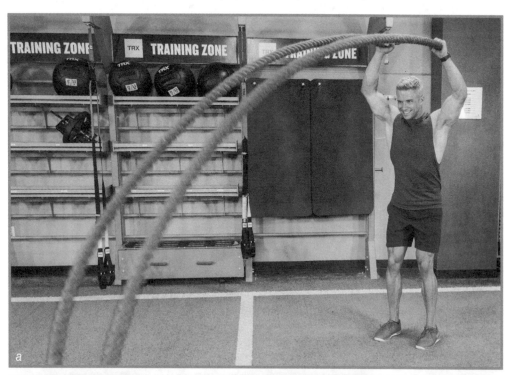

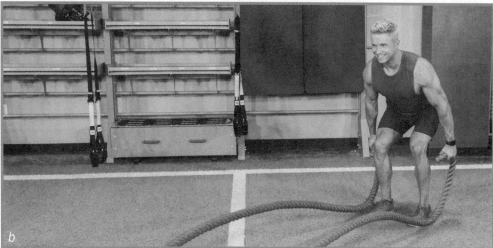

SETUP

Assume a squat stance with feet shoulder-width apart. Hold the ends of the battle ropes low between the legs in a neutral grip with the palms facing in and thumbs on top.

EXECUTION

Explosively stand up from the squat while simultaneously raising arms to approximately shoulder height or higher (see figure *a*). Holding firmly, immediately slam the ropes down as you return to the squat (see figure *b*). Inhale on upward movement and exhale on the downward slam.

Agility Ladder: High-Speed Single- and Double-Foot Contact Runs

SETUP

Stand in an athletic stance with the feet hip-width apart, heels slightly lifted off floor, and knees slightly bent. Face the length of the ladder.

EXECUTION

With either one- or two-foot contact per square, move across the ladder as quickly as possible, swinging the arms to coordinate with foot speed. Stay off of your heels and remain light on your feet. When you reach the end of the ladder, jog back to the starting position. If you performed two-foot contact per square, start the next repetition with the other foot moving first.

BOSU Balance Trainer: Dome Squat Jump

SETUP

Stand tall in a narrow stance on the dome side of a BOSU Balance Trainer with hands at your sides.

EXECUTION

Inhale and squat down, bringing the arms slightly behind you (see figure *a*). Exhale and jump straight up, swinging the arms up next to the head (see figure *b*). Land with control on the dome in a squat position and repeat.

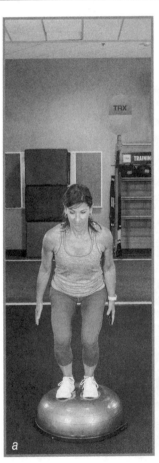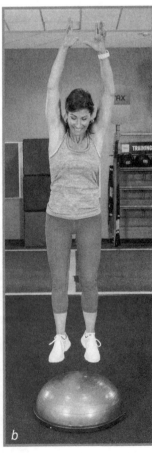

Slam Ball: Double-Arm Slams

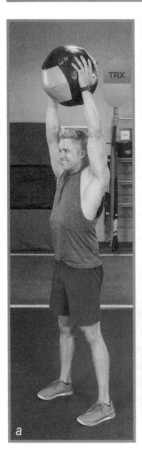 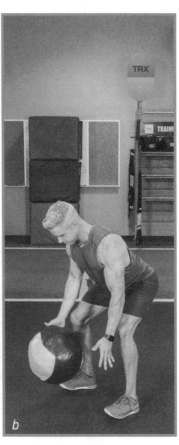

SETUP

Stand tall with the feet shoulder-width apart. Hold a slam ball at chest height with the elbows bent.

EXECUTION

Inhale and bring the ball overhead (see figure *a*). Exhale and powerfully slam the ball onto the ground while moving into a squat (see figure *b*). Pick up the ball and repeat.

Kettlebell: Double-Arm Swings

SETUP

Stand tall with the feet shoulder-width apart and core braced tightly. Hold a kettlebell in both hands, with fingers hooked over the handle.

EXECUTION

Inhale, hinge at the hips, and swing the kettlebell between the legs, keeping the knees soft. Exhale and drive the hips up and forward, maintaining straight arms and allowing the kettlebell to swing level with the shoulders. Keep the core braced and the neck in a neutral position. Return the kettlebell between the legs in an arc and repeat. Focus on the fast, explosive hip drive to swing the kettlebell. Arms do not do the lifting; all the force should come from the lower body.

Battle Ropes: Alternating Waves With Jump Lunge

SETUP

Stand in a split stance lunge with the knees bent. Hold the ends of the battle ropes in a neutral grip with the palms facing in and thumbs on top. The arms are low and the elbows are slightly bent.

EXECUTION

Jump up explosively, switching legs in a lunge while performing small alternating waves with the ropes (see figures *a-c*). Continue for reps or time. Maintain a continuous breath.

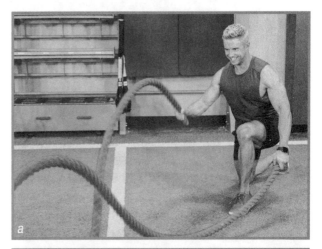

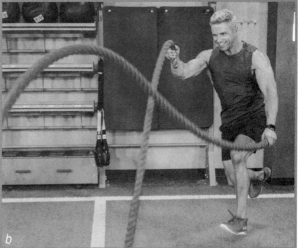

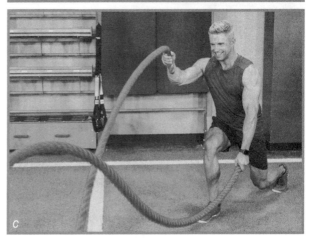

Agility Ladder: Lateral Run-Throughs

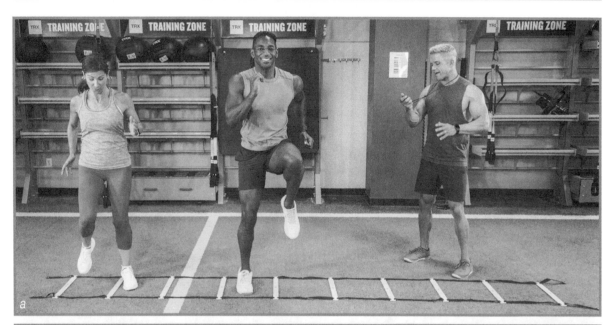

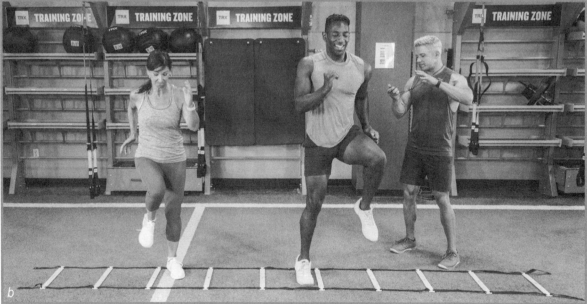

SETUP

Stand in an athletic ready position side-on to an agility ladder with feet hip-width apart and knees slightly bent.

EXECUTION

Moving laterally across the ladder, step in with both feet, then advance to the next square. Stay in the athletic stance and move lightly on the balls of the feet with heels slightly lifted (see figures *a* and *b*). When you reach the end of the ladder, jog back to the starting position and repeat on the other side.

BOSU Balance Trainer: Burpee Push-Ups With Platform Side Up

SETUP

Stand tall with the abdominals engaged and feet shoulder-width apart behind a BOSU Balance Trainer, platform side up.

EXECUTION

Squat down and place the hands on the side edges of the platform. Jump or walk back into a plank position, then perform a push-up on the toes or knees. Jump or walk back to a squat position. Stand up and repeat. Maintain a continuous breath.

Kettlebell: Alternating Single-Arm Swings

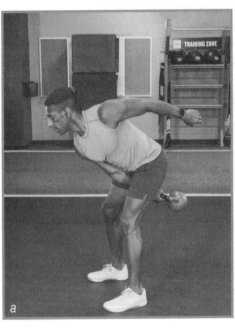 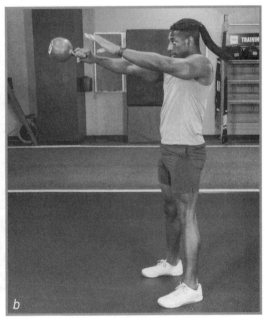

SETUP

Stand tall with the core engaged tightly and feet shoulder-width apart. Hold a kettlebell in one hand with fingers hooked over the handle.

EXECUTION

Inhale, hinge at the hips, and swing the kettlebell between the legs, keeping the knees soft (see figure *a*). Exhale and drive the hips up and forward, maintaining a straight arm and allowing the kettlebell to swing level with the shoulders (see figure *b*). When the kettlebell reaches shoulder height, exchange to the other hand before allowing the kettlebell to swing down. Keep the core braced and the neck in a neutral position. Return the kettlebell between the legs in an arc. Alternate arms for time or repetitions.

Battle Ropes: Alternating Waves

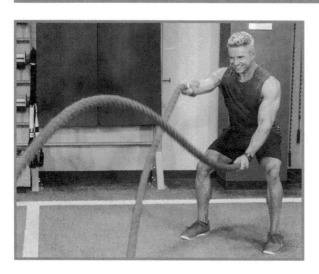

SETUP

Stand in a half squat with feet about shoulder-width apart. Hold the battle ropes in a neutral grip. Contract the core and keep the spine erect.

EXECUTION

Alternating the arms, lift and slam rope down to create waves while maintaining perfect posture and alignment (see figure). Maintain a continuous breath.

Suspension: Inverted Rows

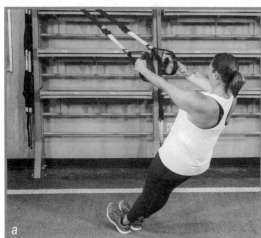

a

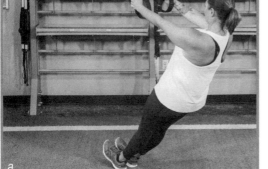

b

SETUP

Stand tall facing the attachment point of a suspension system. Hold the handles with arms fully extended and shoulders flexed, with the palms facing inwards. Keep a rigid body position with a slight lean back (see figure *a*). The closer the feet are to the attachment point and the more the body is reclined, the more challenging the exercise.

EXECUTION

Exhale and pull the body upwards, maintaining a perfect straight line from the heels to the head (see figure *b*). Pull the elbows into the sides of the rib cage, keeping the palms of the hands facing inwards. Pull the shoulder blades together. Inhale and slowly extend arms, lowering the body back to the starting position.

Battle Ropes: Grappler Throws

SETUP

Stand in a half squat with feet shoulder-width apart. Hold the battle ropes in a neutral grip with hands together to one side of the body. Keep the core contracted and the spine erect.

EXECUTION

Inhale and raise explosively out of the squat while powerfully bringing arms up in an arc. Drop back into the half squat and slam the ropes down to the other side of the body while exhaling (see figures *a-c*). Repeat side to side for time or reps.

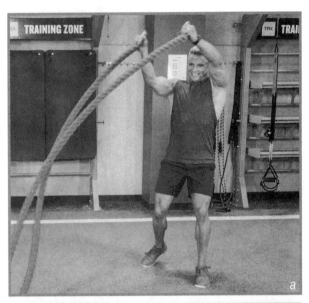

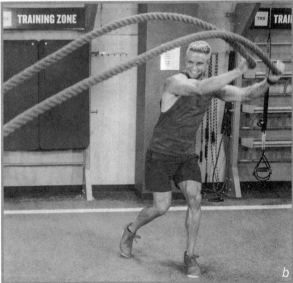

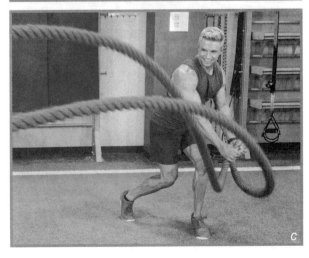

Suspension: Power Pull-Up

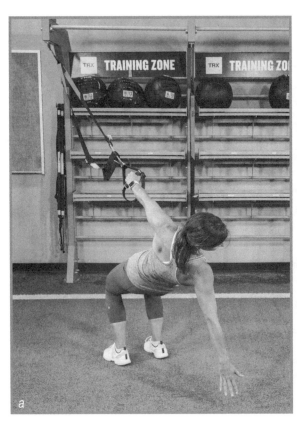
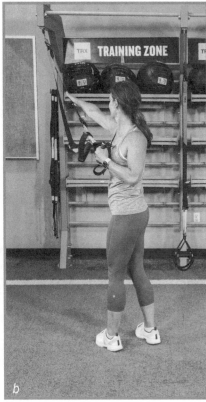

SETUP

Loop the handles of the suspension trainer to create a single stable strap. Hold the strap in one hand and extend the arm. Reach the other arm and hand toward the floor, rotating the body and squatting the hips and knees slightly (see figure *a*). Keep a rigid body position with a slight lean back. The closer the feet are to the attachment point and the more the body is reclined, the more challenging the exercise.

EXECUTION

Exhale and pull the body upwards while rotating the torso, reaching the opposite hand up towards the suspension strap (see figure *b*). Keep the knees bent and the feet shoulder-width apart. Inhale and slowly lower towards the floor again. Repeat for time or reps, then perform on the other side.

Two-Dumbbell Front and Reverse Lunge

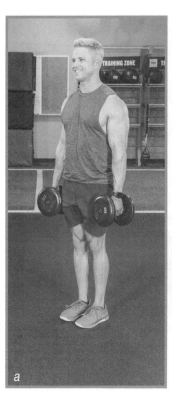
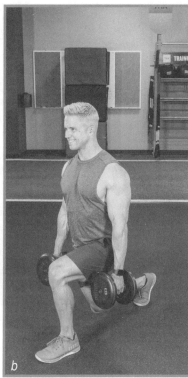
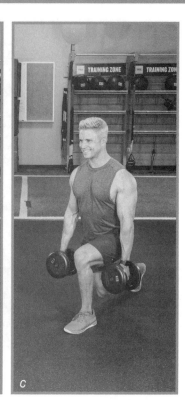

SETUP

Stand tall with the shoulders back and down and the abdominals engaged. Hold a dumbbell in each hand at your sides (see figure *a*).

EXECUTION

Inhale and step the left leg into a front lunge (see figure *b*). Exhale and push back to the starting position. Immediately lunge the right leg backwards into a rear lunge (see figure *c*). Keeping most of the body weight on the left leg, return to the starting position. Alternate for reps or time.

One-Dumbbell Diagonal Chop and Shoulder Press

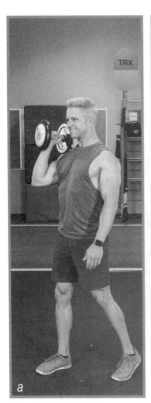
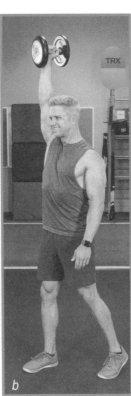
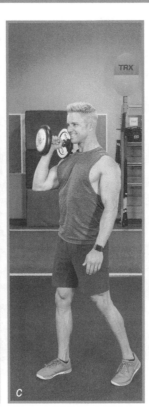
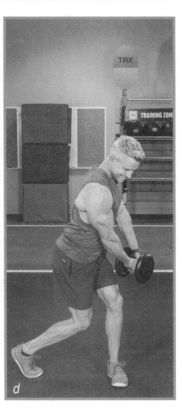

SETUP

Stand with weight shifted to the balls of the feet in a staggered stance with the right leg forward and left leg back. Hold a dumbbell in the right hand at the shoulder with the palm of the hand facing in (see figure *a*).

EXECUTION

Exhale and press the dumbbell overhead, keeping the palm of the hand facing in (see figure *b*). Inhale, bending the elbow to return to start position (see figure *c*). Exhale and place the left hand on top of the right hand, swing the dumbbell towards the left hip, rotate the hips, and swivel the feet to perform a diagonal chop (see figure *d*). Inhale and chop the dumbbell back to the starting position. Repeat for reps or time, then perform on the other side.

Two-Dumbbell Single-Leg Deadlift and Side Lunge

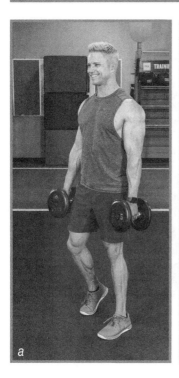

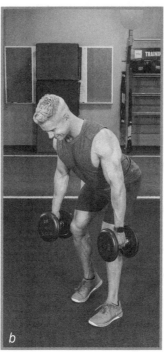

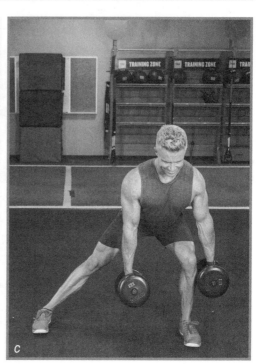

SETUP

Stand tall in a slightly staggered stance with weight on the left foot and the right foot in a "kickstand" position for balance. Hold a dumbbell in each hand at the sides of the body. Keep the abdominals engaged and shoulders down and back (see figure *a*).

EXECUTION

Maintaining most of the weight on the left leg, inhale and hinge at the hip into a single-leg deadlift (see figure *b*). Pull navel to spine to increase core engagement and sustain a neutral spinal position. Exhale and stand back up, keeping the left knee soft. Transferring weight to the right foot, inhale and side lunge to the left (see figure *c*). Keep left toes pointing forward and the feet parallel. Exhale and come back to starting position. Repeat for repetitions or time, then perform on the other side.

Two-Dumbbell Squat and Curl

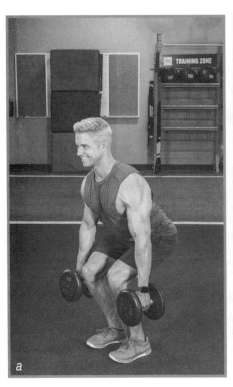
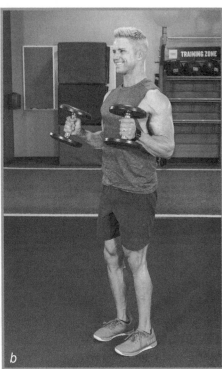

SETUP

Stand tall with feet hip-width apart. Hold a dumbbell in each hand at your sides with abdominals engaged and shoulders down and back.

EXECUTION

Inhale and squat by bending the knees and shifting the hips down and back. Extend the elbows and reach the hands down toward the front of the shins (see figure *a*). Exhale and stand up while simultaneously flexing the elbows, bringing the hands up to the shoulders to perform a biceps curl (see figure *b*). Inhale while lowering dumbbells and repeat.

Two-Dumbbell Crossover Lunge and Side Lunge

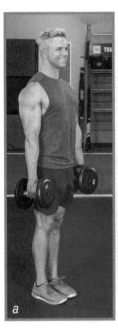 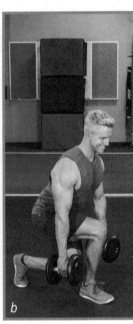 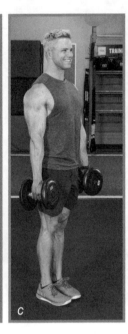 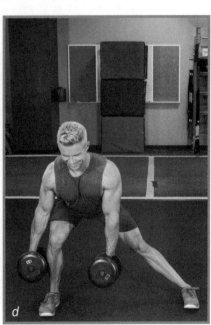

SETUP

Stand tall with the feet together, shoulders down and back, and abdominals engaged. Hold a dumbbell in each hand at your sides (see figure *a*).

EXECUTION

Inhale and step the left leg across and behind the right in a "curtsy" lunge (see figure *b*), maintaining most of the weight on the right leg. Exhale and step feet back together (see figure *c*). Next, inhale and perform a side lunge to the right, keeping the toes straight ahead and feet parallel (see figure *d*). Exhale and push back to the starting position. Repeat for reps or time, then perform on the other side.

Two-Dumbbell Bent-Over Row With Deadlift

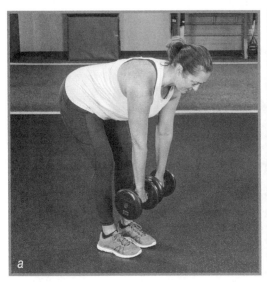 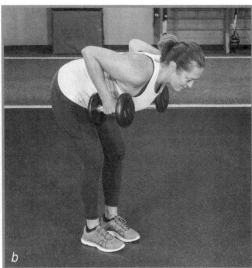

SETUP

Stand tall with the shoulders down and back and the abdominals engaged. Hold a dumbbell in each hand at your sides.

EXECUTION

Keeping knees soft, inhale and hinge forward at the hips, performing a deadlift by reaching the hands toward the shins with extended elbows (see figure *a*). Maintain neutral spine and neck, bracing the core muscles tightly. Staying in the flexed hip position, exhale and perform a dumbbell row, driving elbows toward the ceiling (see figure *b*). Inhale and extend the elbows to lower the hands back to the shins. Finally, exhale and stand back up to the starting position.

Two-Dumbbell Bridge With Triceps Extension

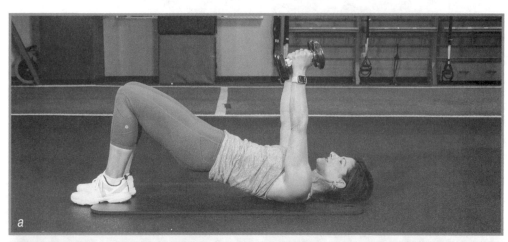

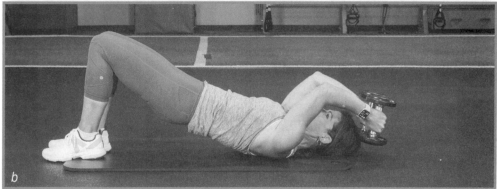

SETUP

Lie in a supine position with the feet flat on the floor hip-width apart and the knees bent. Hold a dumbbell in each hand with arms raised straight above the shoulders. Raise the hips off the floor into a bridge (see figure *a*).

EXECUTION

Simultaneously inhale and lower hips toward the floor while flexing the elbows to lower the dumbbells toward the floor (see figure *b*). The elbows should remain positioned directly above the shoulders. Exhale and extend the elbows, raising the hands and hips at the same time, back to the bridge.

Reverse Lunge to Overhead Press

SETUP

Stand tall with feet together and core braced tightly. With the right hand at the shoulder, hold a dumbbell with the palm of the hand facing in.

EXECUTION

Exhale and press the dumbbell overhead, extending the elbow and keeping the palm of the hand facing in. Hold the arm extended overhead, then inhale and step the left leg back into a reverse lunge, bending both knees and lowering the hips. Maintain a neutral spine and engaged core. Exhale and step forward to bring the feet together. Inhale and lower dumbbell to shoulder. Repeat for reps or time, then perform on the other side.

Push-Ups to Dynamic Beast

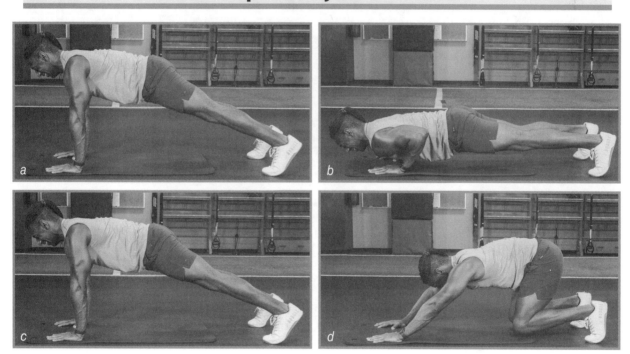

SETUP

Assume a prone plank position with the hands directly under the shoulders, the hips and knees extended, feet shoulder-width apart, and spine neutral (see figure *a*).

EXECUTION

Perform a push-up by inhaling to lower and exhaling to push up (see figures *b* and *c*). The dynamic beast portion of the exercise starts by bending knees, flexing hips towards the heels, and straightening arms (see figure *d*). Finally, exhale and straighten the hips and knees, bringing the body forward until the shoulders are over the hands again. Repeat from the push-up. To modify, perform the push-up from the knees and the dynamic beast from the toes.

Kettlebell Clean and Press

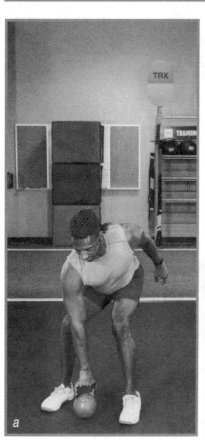
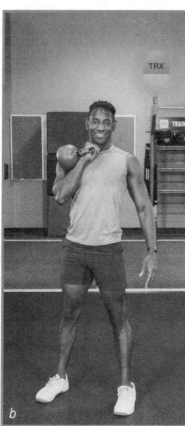
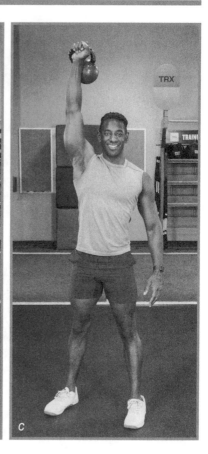

SETUP

Stand tall with the feet shoulder-width apart and the core engaged. Hold a kettlebell in one hand in front of the body with the elbow extended.

EXECUTION

Inhale, bend knees, and drive hips back in a squat (see figure *a*), swinging the kettlebell between the legs. Exhale and powerfully extend the hips and knees while pulling the kettlebell up to the shoulder, "cleaning" it (see figure *b*). "Rack" the kettlebell against the shoulder. Inhale and exhale to perform a shoulder press, pushing the kettlebell directly up, flexing the shoulder and extending the elbow (see figure *c*). Ideally the elbow should be close to the ear. Inhale and lower the kettlebell back to the "rack." Punch the kettlebell forward and away from the body, swinging it back between the legs to repeat.

Kettlebell Goblet Squat

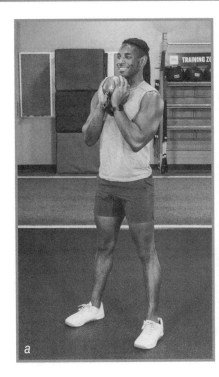 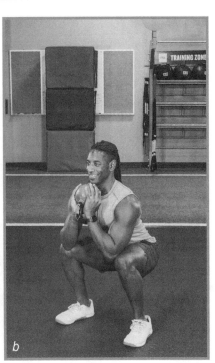

SETUP

Stand tall with feet shoulder-width apart and toes slightly turned out. Hold a kettlebell upside down in both hands at the chest level, shoulders pressed down away from the ears, elbows close to the sides of the body (see figure *a*).

EXECUTION

Inhale and squat down by flexing the hips and knees while sitting the hips back (see figure *b*). Keep spine neutral and erect and brace the core tightly. Exhale and stand back up to the starting position.

Kettlebell Push Press

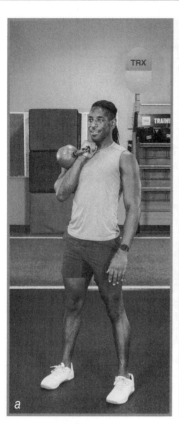
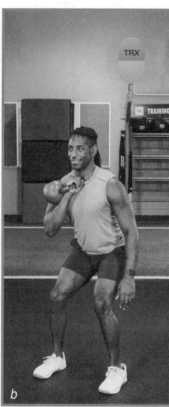
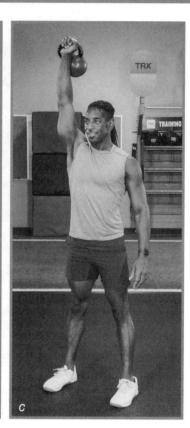

SETUP

Stand tall with feet shoulder-width apart and the core engaged. Hold a kettlebell in the rack position in one hand (see figure *a*).

EXECUTION

Inhale and sit back in a quarter squat, lowering hips and flexing knees slightly (see figure *b*). Exhale and drive up powerfully through the hips, straightening the arms and extending the knees while propelling the kettlebell overhead (see figure *c*). The elbow should finish extended close to the ear, with hand stacked directly above the shoulder. Inhale, then lower the kettlebell back to the rack position. Repeat for reps or time, then perform on the other side.

Mountain Climber

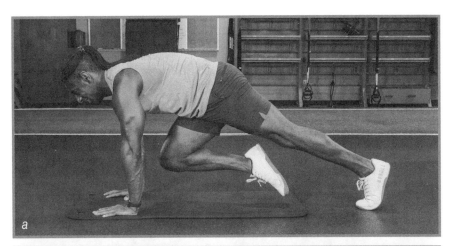

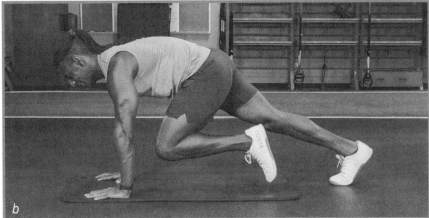

SETUP

Assume a prone plank position, with the hands directly under the shoulders, the hips and knees extended, and the spine long and neutral.

EXECUTION

Lift the right foot off the floor and flex the hip and knee, pulling the knee into the chest (see figure *a*). In a running motion, switch the legs, so the left knee pulls in as the right leg extends out (see figure *b*). Alternate quickly for reps or time. Maintain a continuous breath.

Spiderman Plank

SETUP

Assume a high prone plank position with the knees extended and the core braced tightly. The hands are directly under the shoulders with the elbows extended and the spine neutral.

EXECUTION

Lift the right foot off the floor, flex the knee, and abduct the hip, bringing the knee to the outside of the right elbow. Return the foot to the starting position and repeat on the other side. Maintain a continuous breath.

Super Band Pull-Up

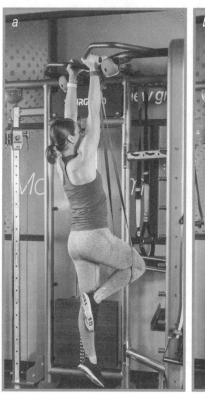 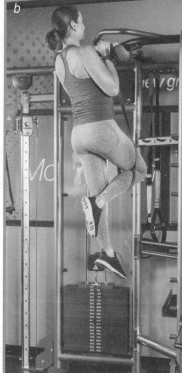

SETUP

Loop a super band through a chin-up bar. Hold the chin-up bar in an overhand grip and place one knee into the band to assist holding the body weight. Extend the elbows and hang from the bar, with one knee supported by the band (see figure *a*).

EXECUTION

While exhaling, pull the body up toward the chin-up bar, until the shoulders are level with the hands (see figure *b*). Inhale and slowly lower the body back down to the starting position.

Suspension: Supine Hamstring Curl

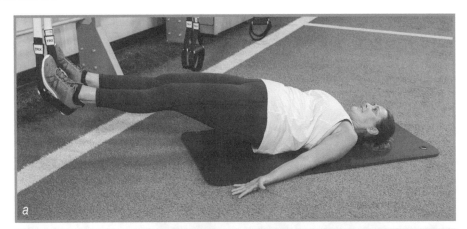

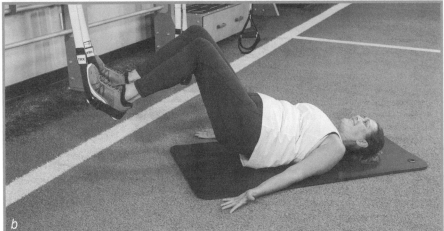

SETUP

Sit on floor in front of suspension system, with the straps adjusted to about 10 inches (20 cm) above the floor. Place the heels into the straps and lie supine with legs extended and straps perpendicular to the floor. The arms are on the floor close to the body, with palms of the hands facing upwards.

EXECUTION

Raise the hips off the floor into a long lever bridge, keeping knees soft (see figure *a*). While exhaling, flex the knees and pull feet towards your hips while keeping the hips raised off the floor (see figure *b*). Inhale, extend the knees to almost full extension, and repeat. If necessary, lower the hips back to the floor between reps for a rest. Maintain a continuous breath.

Sled Push

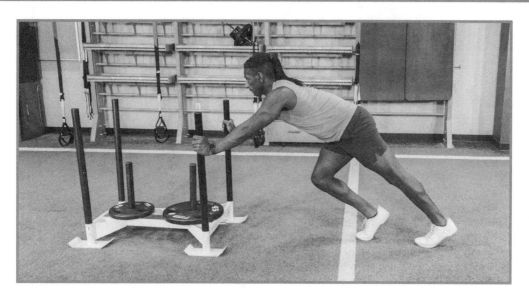

SETUP

Stand behind a sled and hold the bars with the hips flexed forward, core engaged, and spine reasonably neutral (minimal spinal flexion). Load the sled according to the strength of the participant. The load may need to be adjusted for different individuals; this allows for progressions and regressions.

EXECUTION

Taking medium-length strides, push the sled forward, focusing on using the large muscles in the legs and hips (see figure). Maintain good core control by bracing the abdominals and pulling the navel towards the spine. Maintain a continuous breath.

Medicine Ball Russian Twist

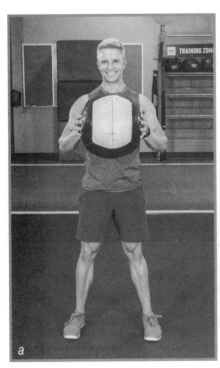 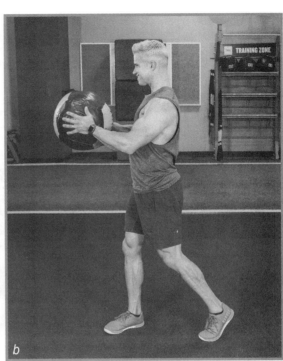

SETUP

Stand tall with feet shoulder-width apart. Hold a medicine ball in front of the body with both hands (see figure *a*). Brace the core by pulling the navel towards the spine.

EXECUTION

Swing to the right, swiveling the left foot and rotating the hips (see figure *b*). Use momentum to rotate from side to side, moving the body as an integrated whole with the hips and feet moving together. Maintain a continuous breath.

Alternating Dome Lunge

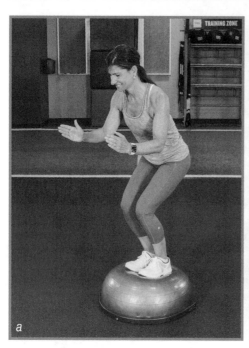 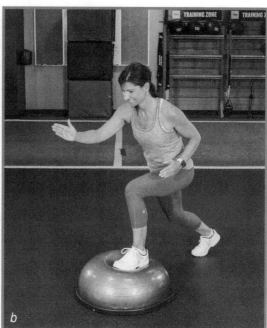

SETUP

Stand tall on the dome side of the BOSU Balance Trainer with feet about hip-width apart, knees soft, and core braced tightly (see figure *a*).

EXECUTION

Inhale and bring right the leg back into a rear lunge (see figure *b*). Exhale and step back up to the start position. Repeat on the other side, alternating for reps or time. To decrease the balance challenge, start on the floor and lunge forward onto the BOSU dome, then bring both feet back together on the floor.

Side-to-Side Squat Jump and Stick on Top of BOSU

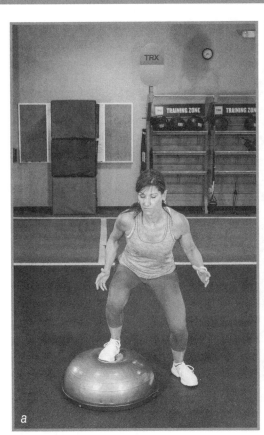 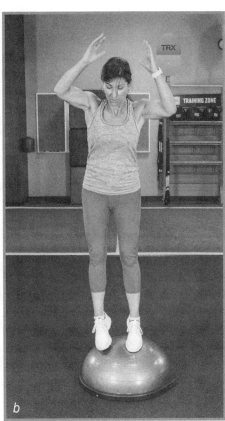

SETUP

Stand tall on the dome side of the BOSU Balance Trainer with the feet hip-width apart, the knees soft, and the core braced.

EXECUTION

Keeping the right foot on the dome, jump the left foot onto the floor to lower into a squat (see figure *a*). Jump back onto the dome to the starting position (see figure *b*). Repeat on the right, alternating for reps or time. To regress, step rather than jump. Keep the core braced and maintain a continuous breath.

Walking Plank

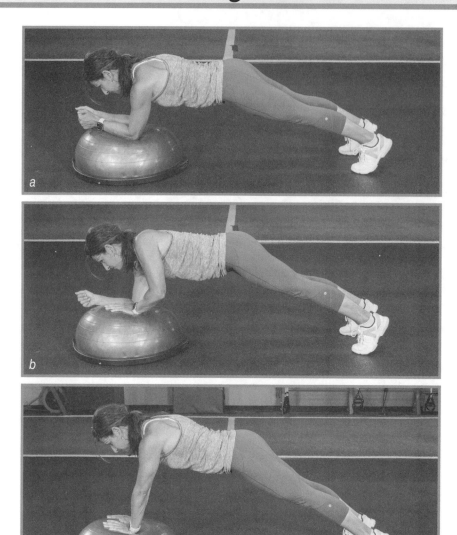

SETUP

Assume a prone plank position with the forearms resting on the dome side of a BOSU Balance Trainer (see figure *a*). The torso is straight with the spine neutral, core braced tightly, and knees extended.

EXECUTION

Walk up onto the hands to extend arms into a high plank (see figures *b* and *c*). Hold at the top, then walk back down onto forearms. Repeat, alternating sides for reps or time. To regress, place knees on the floor. Maintain a continuous breath.

Rear Lunge Knee Touch on Top of BOSU

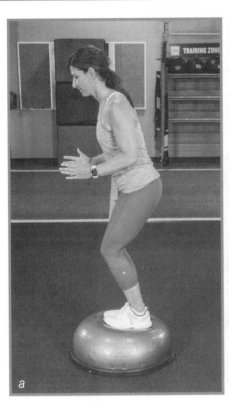
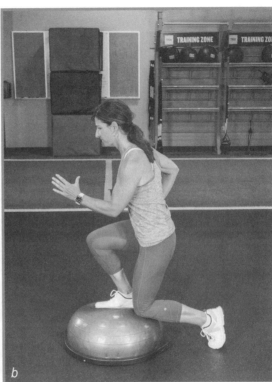

SETUP

Stand tall on the dome side of a BOSU Balance Trainer with the feet about hip-width apart, the knees soft, and the core braced (see figure *a*).

EXECUTION

Lunge the left foot back until the left knee touches the dome (see figure *b*). Bring the left foot back onto the dome. Repeat on the right, alternating for reps or time. To regress, decrease ROM. To progress, add a jump. Keep the core braced and maintain a continuous breath.

SELECTED EXERCISES FOR CHAPTER 14

Split Squat and Bow-and-Arrow Pull

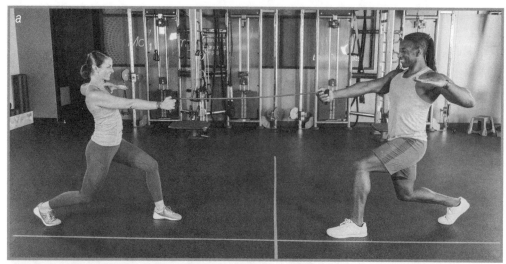

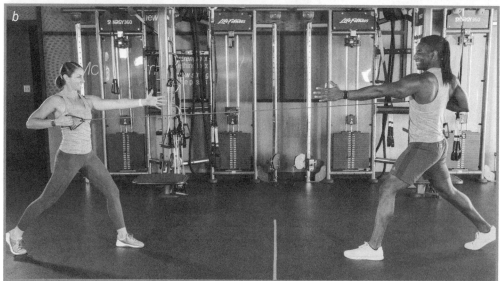

SETUP

Stand facing a partner with the left leg forward in a split squat, each holding the handle of a resistance band in the right hand. Raise the left arm level with the shoulder and pull the elbow back to increase torso rotation like a bow and arrow (see figure *a*). Make sure there is tension on the band from the start of the movement.

EXECUTION

Pull the right hand back and rotate the left hand forward, extending hips and knees to rotate the torso with the arm movement (see figure *b*). Exhale as you raise up and inhale as you lower into the split squat.

Side Plank and Row

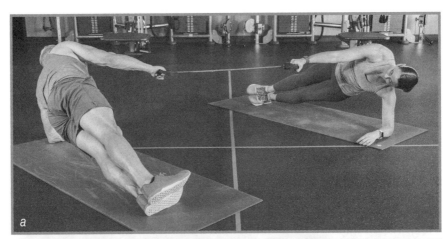

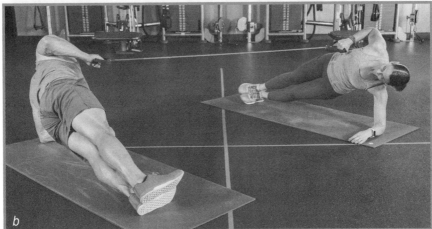

SETUP

Assume a forearm side plank position facing your partner diagonally, each holding the handle of a resistance band in the top hand with the shoulder flexed and the arm extended with light tension (see figure *a*). Brace tightly through the core and maintain a neutral spine.

EXECUTION

Both partners pull the handle toward the side of the rib cage, driving the elbow back (see figure *b*). Maintain a stable side plank position as the rows are performed. To regress, perform the side plank from the knees, in a side bridge.

Squat and High Pull

SETUP

Stand tall with the feet shoulder-width apart, spine neutral, core braced, and shoulders down. Facing a partner, hold the handle of a resistance band in both hands in front of the hips. Stand far enough away from the partner to maintain tension on the band.

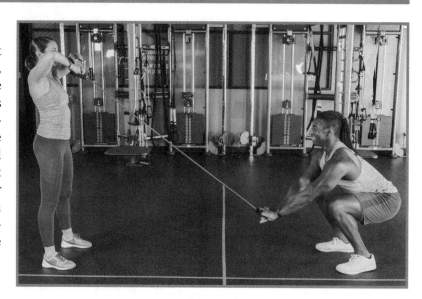

EXECUTION

Partner A squats and pushes the handle of the resistance band down, while simultaneously partner B extends the hips and knees and performs a high pull. Partner A then extends hips and knees and performs a high pull, while partner B squats and pushes the handle of the band down (see figure).

Front Lunge and Chop

SETUP

Stand tall with the feet together facing a partner. Hold the handle of a resistance band in both hands with the arms extended to shoulder height. Stand far enough apart to maintain tension on the band.

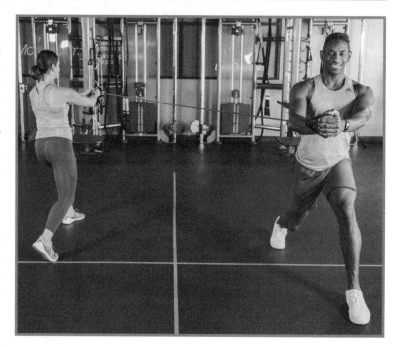

EXECUTION

Both partners pivot and step forward with the left leg while simultaneously chopping horizontally to the left with the resistance band (see figure). Step the left foot back to the starting position and square the body off to the center. Repeat on the right, alternating for reps or time.

Chain-Gang Squat

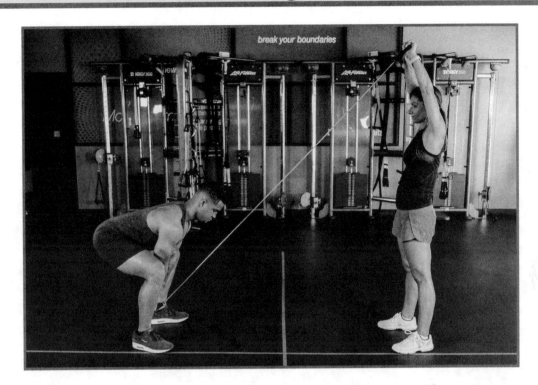

SETUP

Stand tall and face a partner with the feet shoulder-width apart or slightly wider, toes slightly turned out, and core braced tightly. Hold the handle of a resistance band in both hands. Stand far enough apart to maintain tension on the band. The core is braced tightly.

EXECUTION

Partner A squats down and pulls the resistance band between the legs, like a kettlebell swing. Simultaneously, partner B extends the hips and flexes the shoulders, raising the arms overhead (see figure). One person is up while the other is down, like a seesaw.

Chest Press With Front Lunge

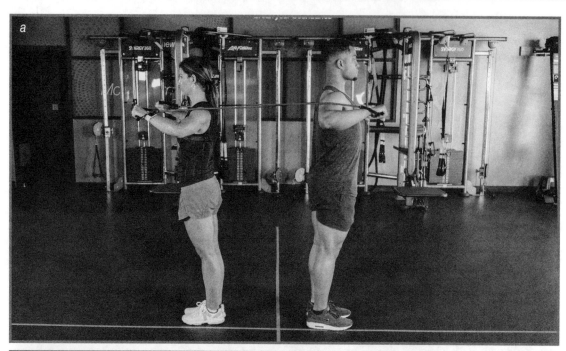

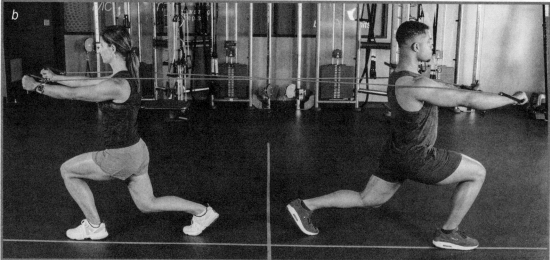

SETUP

Stand tall with feet together facing away from your partner. Loop two resistance bands so each partner is holding the handles of their own resistance band in each hand. The shoulders are abducted so that the hands are directly in front of the shoulders and the band is on top of the arms (see figure *a*). Stand far enough apart to maintain tension on the band.

EXECUTION

Both partners simultaneously step forward into a front lunge while performing a chest press (see figure *b*). Brace the core tightly and exhale while stepping forward. Step the foot back and inhale. Repeat alternating legs.

Side-by-Side Alternating Chop

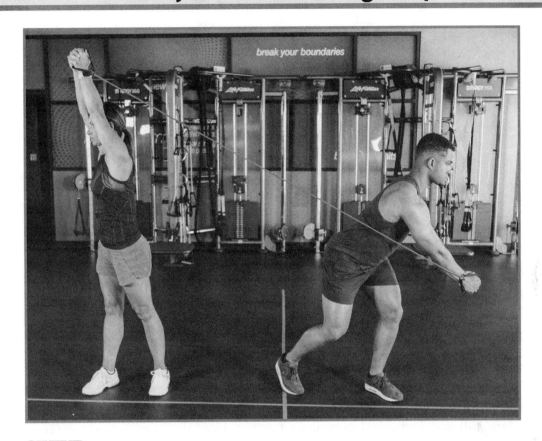

SETUP

Stand side-on to a partner with feet hip-width apart. Hold the handle of a resistance band in both hands with arms extended at shoulder height. Stand far enough apart to maintain tension on the band.

EXECUTION

Partner A performs a high rotation movement away from partner B, while partner B performs a low rotation movement away from partner A (see figure). Both partners return to the starting position. Alternate high and low for reps or time.

Side Lunge With High Pull

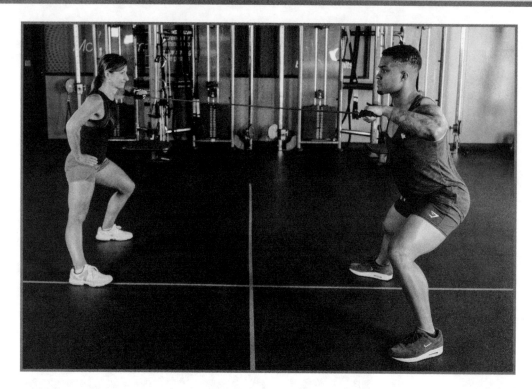

SETUP

Stand tall with feet together facing a partner. Hold the handle of a resistance band in the left hand with arm extended to shoulder height. Stand far enough apart to maintain tension on the band.

EXECUTION

Both partners simultaneously perform a side lunge to the left, keeping feet parallel and sitting back slightly with hips as knees flex. While performing the side lunge, pull the resistance band towards the shoulder, driving the elbow back, to execute a high pull (see figure). Return to the start position and repeat on the right side. Alternate sides for reps or time.

Partner Bicycle

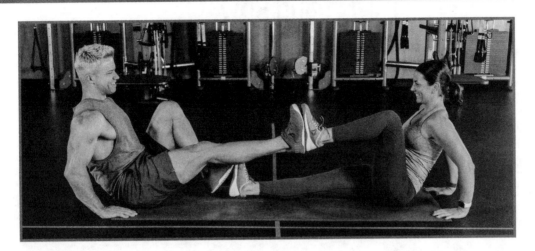

SETUP

Sitting on the floor, face a partner and press the soles of the feet together off the floor in a V-sit. Lean the torso back slightly and place the hands on the floor close to the hips, using the arms to provide support. Sit far enough apart that each person can move through a full ROM.

EXECUTION

Working together, push out one leg and pull the other in, like a bicycle (see figure). Keep the soles of the feet pressed together and move back and forward with the legs. To regress, drop back onto the elbows. To progress, reach the arms out to the sides.

Resistance Band Partner Split Squat and Row

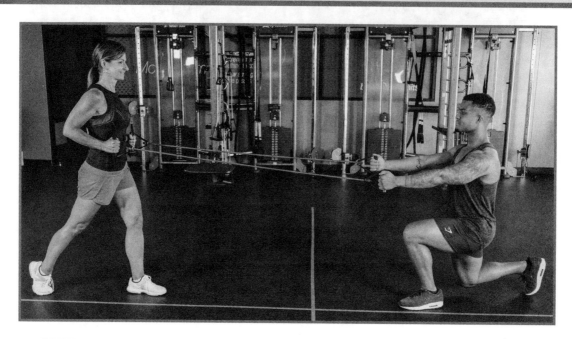

SETUP

In a split squat with arms extended at shoulder height, hold the handles of a resistance band in each hand while facing a partner. Stand far enough apart to maintain tension on the band.

EXECUTION

Taking turns with a partner, exhale and extend the hips and knees into an upright position, simultaneously pulling the elbows in to the rib cage and pushing the shoulder blades back and down (see figure). Inhale and lower to the starting position with control. Repeat for reps or time, then perform the exercise with the opposite leg forward.

Transverse Lunge With Sword Draw

SETUP

Stand tall with the feet together and core braced tightly, facing a partner. Hold the handle of a resistance band in the right hand. Stand far enough apart to maintain tension on the band.

EXECUTION

Exhale and step the right foot back to 4 o'clock, bending the right knee to sink the hips back. Simultaneously, pull the band diagonally to an overhead position with the arm slightly abducted and externally rotated. Keep the left leg fully extended and the foot flat and facing forward (at 12 o'clock). Inhale and return to the starting position. Repeat for reps or time, then perform on the other side.

Suspension Single-Leg Squat and Row

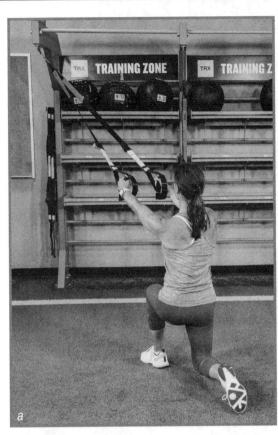 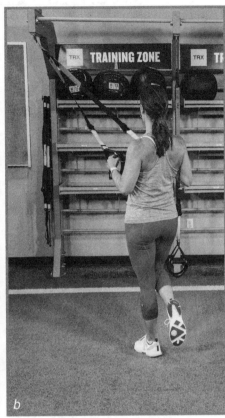

SETUP

Facing the attachment point of a suspension trainer with the handles in each hand, walk the left foot forward to the desired position and dorsiflex the ankle to dig the heel into the floor. Lift the right foot off the floor and raise the leg behind the body, flexing the knee. Squat down with the right leg, extend the elbows and flex the shoulders, and lean back (see figure *a*). The core is braced tightly.

EXECUTION

Exhale and extend the hip and knee of the left leg, coming out of the squat, while simultaneously pulling the body forward and upwards (see figure *b*). Pull the elbows close to the rib cage while drawing the shoulder blades together and down. Inhale and lower back down.

Medicine Ball Front Lunge With Overhead Chop and Rotation

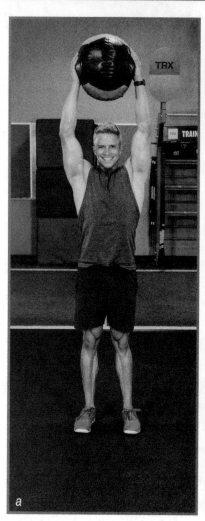

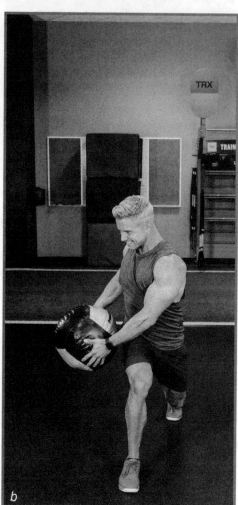

SETUP

Stand tall with the feet about hip-width apart and the elbows extended, holding a medicine ball overhead (see figure *a*). The core is braced tightly to prevent lumbar spinal extension.

EXECUTION

Exhale and lunge the right leg forward while simultaneously chopping the medicine ball down across the right leg (see figure *b*). Inhale and push to starting position while simultaneously chopping the ball back to the overhead position. Repeat on the other side.

Medicine Ball Squat Swing and Toss

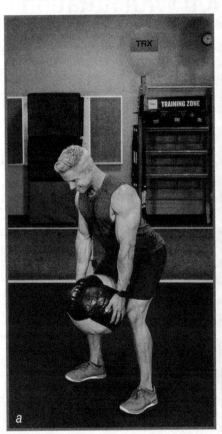
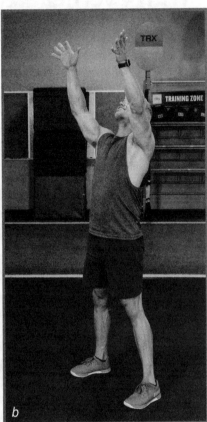

SETUP

Stand tall with the feet shoulder-width apart and the core braced tightly. Hold a medicine ball in both hands in front of the body.

EXECUTION

Inhale and squat down while swinging the ball between the legs, maintaining a neutral spine (see figure *a*). Exhale strongly and swing the ball up while standing up from the squat. At the top of the movement, release the ball into the air, directly overhead (see figure *b*). Catch the ball and repeat the squat, swing, and toss.

Medicine Ball Side Lunge With Overhead Chop With Rotation

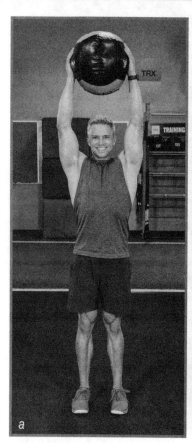
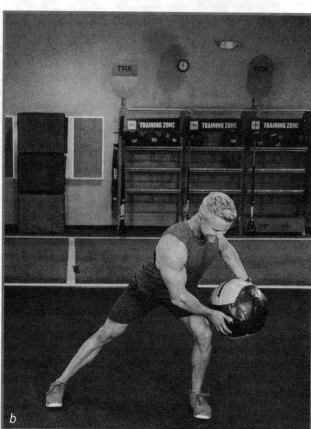

SETUP

Stand tall with the feet together. Hold a medicine ball overhead with the elbows extended (see figure *a*). Brace core strongly to prevent lumbar spinal extension.

EXECUTION

Exhale and lunge to the side with the left foot, simultaneously chopping the ball down to the outside of the left thigh (see figure *b*). Inhale and push back to standing while chopping the ball back overhead. Repeat to the right, alternating for reps or time.

Kettlebell Side Lunge and Swing

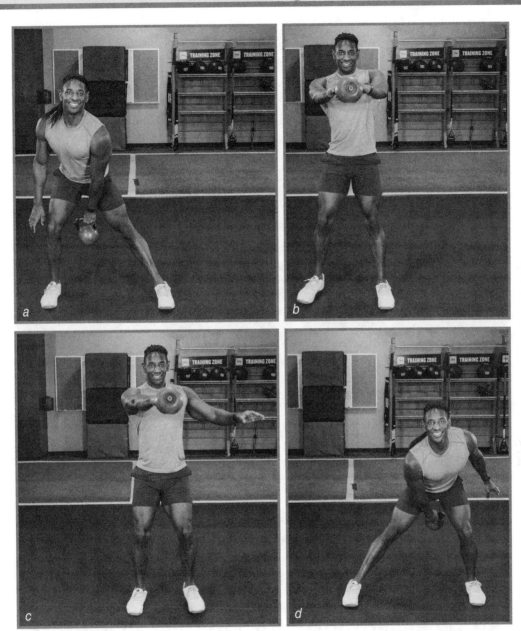

SETUP

Stand tall with the feet together. Hold a kettlebell in the left hand with the arm at the side of the body.

EXECUTION

Inhale and side lunge to the right while swinging the bell between the legs (see figure *a*). Exhale and return to start while swinging the kettlebell back up to shoulder height. Exchange hands at the top of the swing, taking the bell in the right hand (see figures *b* and *c*), then lunge to the left and swing the kettlebell between the legs (see figure *d*). Keep alternating for reps or time.

Medicine Ball Transverse Lunge With Rotation

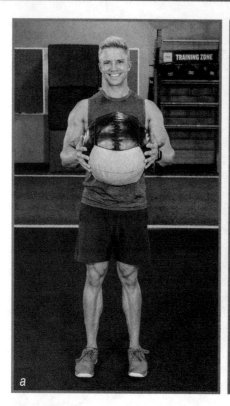 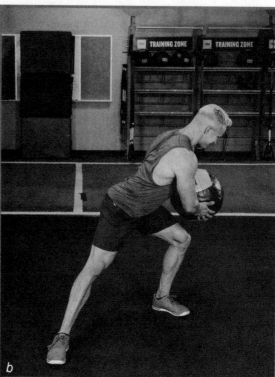

SETUP

Stand tall with the feet together and core braced tightly. Hold a medicine ball in front of the body in both hands with the elbows slightly bent (see figure *a*).

EXECUTION

Rotate to the left, to the right, then back to the left. On the third rotation, step and bend the left knee and hip into a transverse lunge while also chopping the ball to the left (see figure *b*). Return to the starting position. Repeat the three rotations and one lunge on the other side.

Kettlebell Front Lunge and Overhead Press

SETUP

Stand tall with the feet together and the core braced tightly. Hold a kettlebell in the rack position in the right hand.

EXECUTION

Lunge the left leg forward, pressing the kettlebell overhead at the bottom of the lunge. Hold the lunge and lower the kettlebell back to the rack position. Push back to the starting position. Maintain a continuous breath. Repeat for reps or time, then perform on the other side.

Medicine Ball Squat With Reverse Lunge and Overhead Press

SETUP

Stand tall with feet hip-width apart and core braced tightly. Hold a medicine ball in front of the chest with the elbows flexed.

EXECUTION

Inhale and squat down, then exhale and stand to return to the starting position. Inhale and lunge the right leg back, sinking the hips and flexing the knees. Exhale and press the medicine ball overhead at the bottom of the lunge. Inhale and lower the ball back to the chest, then exhale and step the right foot back to the starting position. Repeat the squat, then lunge the left leg back and repeat the overhead press. Keep alternating the lunging leg and perform a squat between each lunge for reps or time.

Kettlebell Windmill

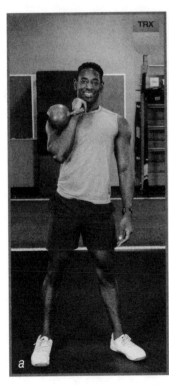 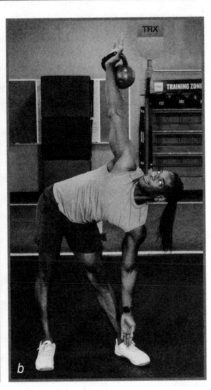

SETUP

Stand tall with the feet slightly more than shoulder-width apart. Rotate the body to an open stance with the left foot externally rotated and the right foot internally rotated. Hold a kettlebell in the rack position in the right hand (see figure *a*).

EXECUTION

Flex at the hips laterally and press the kettlebell up from the rack position, perpendicular to the floor, while reaching the left hand towards the left foot (see figure *b*). Brace the core tightly and focus on keeping the body in the frontal plane. Repeat for reps or time before performing the other side.

Medicine Ball Curtsy Lunge and Ball Bounce

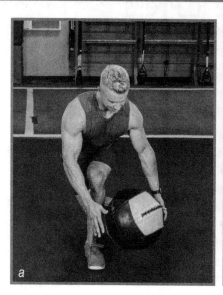

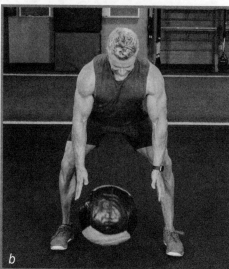

SETUP

Stand tall with the feet hip-width apart. Hold a medicine ball in front of the chest with the elbows flexed.

EXECUTION

Cross the right leg behind the left into a curtsy lunge and simultaneously slam the ball down to bounce it (see figure *a*). Catch it on the way up as you bring the feet together again (see figure *b*). Repeat on the other side, slamming and bouncing the ball on each curtsy lunge.

Kettlebell Racked Front Squat to Reverse Lunge With Overhead Press

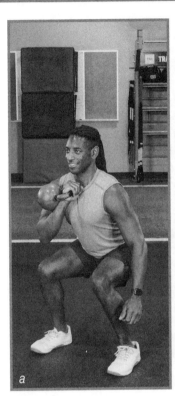
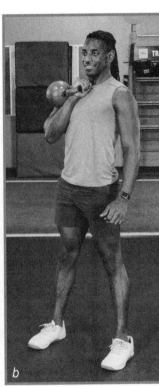
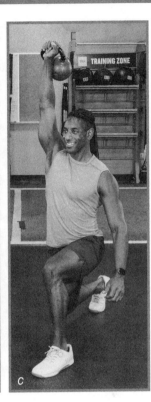

SETUP

Stand tall with feet shoulder-width apart and core braced tightly. Hold a kettlebell in the racked position on the right side.

EXECUTION

Inhale and squat down, maintaining a neutral spine (see figure *a*). Exhale and return to a standing position (see figure *b*). Lunge the right leg back, performing an overhead press at the bottom of the lunge (see figure *c*). Lower the kettlebell, stand back up, and perform another squat. Repeat for reps before performing the other side. To progress, try a heavier bell and press the kettlebell overhead before performing the lunge, or stand back up from the lunge before lowering the kettlebell back to the rack for the squat.

REFERENCES

Chapter 1

Firestone, M.J., Yi, S.S., Bartley, K.F., & Eisenhower, D.L. (2015). Perceptions and the role of group exercise among New York City adults, 2010-2011: An examination of interpersonal factors and leisure-time physical activity. *Preventive Medicine, 72*, 50-55. doi:10.1016/j.ypmed.2015.01.001

Thompson, W. (2006). Worldwide survey reveals fitness trends for 2007. *ACSM's Health & Fitness Journal, 10*(6), 8-14. doi:10.1249/01.FIT.0000252519.52241.39

Thompson, W. (2016). Worldwide survey of fitness trends for 2017. *ACSM's Health & Fitness Journal, 20*(6), 8-17. doi:10.1249/FIT.0000000000000252

Yoke, M.M., & Kennedy, C. (2003). *Functional exercise progressions.* Monterey, CA: Coaches Choice.

Chapter 2

American College of Sports Medicine. (2012). *ACSM's health/fitness facility standards and guidelines* (4th ed.). Champaign, IL: Human Kinetics.

Hobson, A. (Ed.), (2004). *The Oxford dictionary of difficult words.* Oxford University Press.

International Health, Racquet and Sportsclub Association. (2005). *IHRSA's guide to club membership and conduct.* Boston, MA.

Chapter 4

Fehr, E., & Gächter, S. (2000). Fairness and retaliation: The economics of reciprocity. *Journal of Economic Perspectives, 14*(3), 159-181.

Kennedy, D.S. (2013). *No B.D. direct marketing: The ultimate no holds barred kick butt take no prisoners direct marketing for non-direct marketing businesses.* Irvine, CA: Entrepreneur Press.

Vogel, Amanda. *FitnessTestDrive.com*

Chapter 5

American College of Sports Medicine (ACSM). (2017). *ACSM's guidelines for exercise testing and prescription* (10th ed.). Philadelphia: Lippincott, Williams & Wilkins.

American Council on Exercise (ACE). (2014). *ACE personal trainer manual* (5th ed.). San Diego, CA.

Blair, S.N., Kohl, H.W. III, Barlow, C.E., Paffenbarger, R.S. Jr., Gibbons, L.W., & Macera, C.A. (1995). Changes in physical fitness and all-cause mortality. A prospective study of healthy and unhealthy men. *Journal of the American Medical Association, 273*(14), 1093-1098.

Bray, G.A. (2004). Don't throw the baby out with the bath water. *American Journal of Clinical Nutrition, 70*(3), 347-349.

Despres, J.P. (2012) Body fat distribution and risk of cardiovascular disease: An update. *Circulation, 126*(10), 1301-1313.

Lohman, T.G. (1981). Skinfolds and body density and their relation to body fatness: A review. *Human Biology, 53*(2), 181-225.

McGill, S. (2015). *Low back disorders: Evidence-based prevention and rehabilitation* (3rd ed.). Champaign, IL: Human Kinetics.

Ostechega, Y., Fryar C., Nwankwo, T., & Nguyen, D. (2020). Hypertension prevalence among adults aged 18 and over: United States, 2017-2018. In *Centers for disease control and prevention: National center for health statistics data brief 364.*

Chapter 6

Fredrickson, Barbara. 2009. *Positivity: groundbreaking research reveals how to embrace the hidden strength of positive emotions, overcome negativity and thrive.* New York, NY. Penguin Random House.

Karageorghis, C.I., Jones, L., Priest, D.L., Akers, R.I., Clarke, A., Perry, J.M., Reddick, B.T., Bishop, D.T., & Lim, H.B. (2011). Revisiting the relationship between exercise heart rate and music tempo preference. *American Alliance for Health Physical Education Recreation and Dance: Research Quarterly for Exercise and Sport, 82*(2), 274-284.

Prochaska & DiClemente. (2014). *Detailed overview of the transtheoretical model.*

Velicer, W. F, Prochaska, J. O., Fava, J. L., Norman, G. J., & Redding, C. A. (1998). Smoking cessation and stress management: Applications of the transtheoretical model of behavior change. *Homeostasis, 38,* 216-233.

Seligman, Martin E.P., Ernst, Randall M., Gillham, Jane, Reivich, Karen, & Linkins, Mark. (2009). Positive education: positive psychology and classroom interventions. *Oxford Review of Education, 35*(3), 293-311.

Chapter 7

Boutcher, S.H. (2008). Attentional processes and sport performance. In T. S. Horn (Ed.), *Advances in sport psychology* (pp. 325-338, 467-470). Champaign, IL: Human Kinetics.

Murphy, S.M., and K.A. Martin. (2002). The use of imagery in sport. In T. S. Horn (Ed.), *Advances in sport psychology* (pp. 405-39). Champaign, IL: Human Kinetics.

Bacon, S.J. (1974).Arousal and the range of cue utilization. *Journal of Experimental Psychology, 102*(1), 81-7. doi:10.1037/h0035690

Easterbrook, J.A. (1959). The effects of emotion on cue utilization and the organization of behavior. *Psychological Review, 66,* 183-201. doi:10.1037/h0047707.

Nideffer, R.M., M.S. Sagal, M. Lowry, & J. Bond. (2001). Identifying and developing world class performers. In Gershon Tenenbaum (Ed.), *The practice of sport psychology, fitness information technology* (pp. 129-144).

Wachtel, P.L. (1967). Conceptions of broad and narrow attention. *Psychological Bulletin, 68*(6): 417-429. doi:10.1037/h0025186.

Chapter 8

Bryant, C.X., D.J. Green, S. Newton-Merrill, American Council on Exercise. (2013). *ACE health coach manual : the ultimate guide to wellness, fitness, and lifestyle change.* San Diego, CA: American Council on Exercise.

Dungy, T. (2010). *The mentor leader: Secrets to building people and teams that win consistently.* Carol Stream, IL: Tyndale Momentum Publishers.

Chapter 9

McGill, S. (2002). *Low back disorders.* (3rd ed.). Champaign, IL: Human Kinetics.

De Souza, E.O., V. Tricoli, J. Rauch, M.R. Alvarez, G. Laurentino, A.Y. Aihara, F.N. Cardoso, H. Roschel, & C. Ugrinowitsch. (2018). Different patterns in muscular strength and hypertrophy adaptations in untrained individuals undergoing nonperiodized and periodized strength regimens. *J Strength Cond Res, 32*(5), 1238-1244. doi:10.1519/JSC.0000000000002482.

Pelzer, T., B. Ulrich, and M. Pfeiffer. (2017). Periodization effects during short-term resistance training with equated exercise variables in females. *European Journal of Applied Physiology, 177,* 441-454. doi:10.1007/s00421-017-3544-x.

Williams, T.D., D.V. Tolusso, M.V. Fedewa, & M.R. Esco. (2017). Comparison of periodized and non-periodized resistance training on maximal strength: A meta-analysis. *Sports Med, 47,* 2083-100. doi:10.1007/s40279-017-0734-y.

McNamara, J.M., & D.J. Stearne. (2010). Flexible nonlinear periodization in a beginner college weight training class. *J Strength Cond Res, 24*(1): 17-22. doi:10.1519/JSC.0b013e3181bc177b.

Evans, J.W. (2019). Periodized resistance training for enhancing skeletal muscle hypertrophy and strength: A mini-review. *Front Physiol, 23.* doi:10.3389/fphys.2019.00013.

Kok, L., P.W. Hamer, & D.J. Bishop. (2009). Enhancing muscular qualities in untrained women: linear versus undulating periodization. *Med Sci Sports Exerc, 41*(9). 1797-1807. doi:10.1249/MSS.0b013e3181a154f3.

Grgic, J., P. Mikulic, H. Podnar, & Z. Pedisic. (2017). Effects of linear and daily undulating periodized resistance training programs on measures of muscle hypertrophy: A systematic review and meta-analysis. *PeerJ, 5.* doi:10.7717/peerj.3695.

Evans, J.W. (2019). Periodized resistance training for enhancing skeletal muscle hypertrophy and strength: A mini-review. *Front. Physiol, 23.* doi:10.3389/fphys.2019.00013.

Chapter 10

Borsheim, E., & Bahr, R. (2003). Effect of exercise intensity, duration and mode on post-exercise oxygen consumption. *Sports Medicine, 33*(14), 1037-1060.

Boutcher, S.H. (2011). High-intensity intermittent exercise and fat loss. *Journal of Obesity.* doi:10.1155/2011/868305

Coggan, A., A. Hunter, & S. McGregor. (2019). *Training and Racing with a Power Meter, Third Edition.* Boulder, CO: Velo Press.

Dalleck, L.C., & Kravitz, L. (2003). Optimize endurance training. *IDEA Personal Trainer, 14*(1), 36-42.

Gibala, M.J., Little, J.P., Macdonald, M.J., & Hawley, J.A. (2012). Physiological adaptations to low-volume, high-intensity interval training in health and disease. *Journal of Physiology, 590*(5), 1077-1084. doi:10.1113/jphysiol.2011.22472

Girard, O., Mendez-Villaneuva, A., & Bishop, D. (2011). Repeated-sprint ability—part I: Factors contributing to fatigue. *Sports Medicine, Aug 1, 41*(8), 673-694.

Iaia, F.M., Rampinini, E., & Bangsbo, J. (2009). High-intensity training in football. *International Journal of Sports Physiology and Performance, 4*(3), 291-306. doi:10.1123/ijspp.4.3.291

Kaminski, L.A., & Whaley, M.H. (1993). Effect of internal type exercise on excess post-exercise oxygen consumption (EPOC) in obese and normal-weight women. *Medicine in Exercise, Nutrition and Health, 2,* 106-111.

Kelleher, A.R., Hackney, K.J., Fairchild, T.J., Keslacy, S., & Ploutz-Snyder, L.L. (2010). The metabolic costs of reciprocal supersets vs. traditional resistance exercise in young recreationally active adults. *Journal of Strength and Conditioning Research, 24*(4), 1043-1051.

Kessler, H.S., Sisson, S.B., & Short, K.R. (2012). The potential for high-intensity interval training to reduce cardiometabolic disease risk. *Sports Medicine, 42*(6), 489-509. doi:10.2165/11630910-000000000-00000

Kravitz, L. (2014). Metabolic effects of HIIT. *IDEA Fitness Journal, 11*(5), 16-18.

McGehee, J.C., Tanner, C.J., & Hourmar, J.A. (2005). A comparison of methods for estimating the lactate threshold. *Journal of Strength and Conditioning Research, 19*(3), 553-558.

Perry, C.G.R., Heigenhauser, G.J.F., Bonen, A., & Spriet, L.L. (2008). High-intensity aerobic interval training increases fat and carbohydrate metabolic capacities in human skeletal muscle. *Applied Physiology, Nutrition, and Metabolism, 33,* 1112-11123.

Piras, A., Persiani, M., Damiani, N., Perazzolo, M., & Raffi, M. (2015). Peripheral heart action (PHA) training as a valid substitute to high intensity interval training to improve resting cardiovascular changes and autonomic adaptation. *European Journal of Applied Physiology, 115*(4), 763-773.

Plisk, S. (1991). Anaerobic metabolic conditioning: A brief review of theory, strategy and practical application. *Journal of Strength and Conditioning Research,* 22-34.

Robergs, R.A., Ghiasvand, F., & Parker, D. (2004). Biochemistry of exercise-induced metabolic acidosis. *American Journal of Physiology: Regulatory, Integrative, and Comparative Physiology, 287*(3), R502-R516.

Tabata, I., Nishimura, K., Kouzaki, M., Hirai, Y., Ogita, F., Miyachi, M., et al. (1996). Effects of moderate-intensity endurance and high-intensity intermittent training on anaerobic capacity and VO2max. *Medicine and Science in Sports and Exercise, 28*(10), 1327-1330. doi:10.1097/00005768-199610000-00018

Tremblay, A., Simoneau, J.A., & Bouchard, C. (1994). Impact of exercise intensity on body fatness and skeletal muscle metabolism. *Metabolism, 43*(7), 814-818. doi:10.1016/0026-0495(94)90259-3

Turner, A. (2011). The science and practice of periodization: A brief review. *Strength and Conditioning Journal, 33*(1), 34-46. doi: 10.1519/SSC.0b013e3182079cdf.

Vella, C. (2004). Exercise after-burn: Research update. *IDEA Fitness Journal, 1*(5), 42-47.

Zuhl, M., & Kravitz, L. (2012). HIIT vs. continuous endurance training: Battle of the aerobic titans. *IDEA Fitness Journal, 9*(2), 34.

Chapter 11

Beedle, B.B., & Mann, C.L. (2007). A comparison of two warm-ups on joint range of motion. *Journal of Strength and Conditioning Research, 21*(3), 776-779.

Fletcher, G.F., Balady, G.J., Amsterdam, E.A., Chaitman, B., Eckel, R., Fleg, J., et al. (2001). Exercise standards for testing and training: A statement for healthcare professionals from the American Heart Association. *Circulation, 104*(14), 1694-1740.

Page, P. (2012). Current concepts in muscle stretching for exercise and rehabilitation. *International Journal of Sports Physical Therapy, 7*(1), 109-119.

Simic, L., Sarabon, N., & Markovic, G. Does pre-exercise static stretching inhibit maximal muscular performance? A meta-analytical review. *Scandinavian Journal of Medicine and Science in Sports,* 23(2), 131-148.

Herbert, R.D., and Gabriel, Michael. (2002). Effects of stretching before and after exercising on muscle soreness and risk of injury: Systematic review. *BMJ,* (325), 468.

Chaabene, H., Behm, D.G., Negra, Y., Granacher, U. (2019). Acute effects of static stretching on muscle strength and power: an attempt to clarify previous caveats. *Front Physiol.* doi:10.3389/fphys.2019.01468

Chapter 12

American College of Sports Medicine (ACSM). (2017). *ACSM's guidelines for exercise testing and prescription* (10th ed.). Philadelphia, PA: Lippincott, Williams & Wilkins.

American Council on Exercise (ACE). (2014). *ACE personal trainer manual* (5th ed.). San Diego, CA.

Foster, C., Wright, G., Battista, R.A., & Porcari, J.P. (2009). Training in the aging athlete. *Current Sports Medicine Reports, 6.* 200-206. doi: 10.1007/s11932-007-0029-4

Chapter 13

Boutcher, S.H. (2011). High-intensity intermittent exercise and fat loss. *Journal of Obesity.* doi:10.1155/2011/868305

Kessler, H.S., Sisson, S.B., & Short, K.R. (2012). The potential for high-intensity interval training to reduce cardiometabolic disease risk. *Sports Medicine, 42*(6): 489-509. doi:10.2165/11630910-000000000-00000

INDEX

ABOUT THE AUTHOR

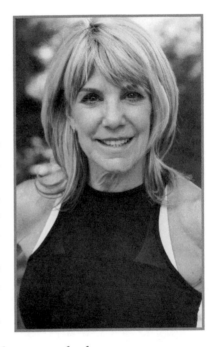

Keli Roberts is a world-renowned fitness educator and trainer. She is certified by the American College of Sports Medicine as an exercise physiologist (ACSM-EP). She is an ACE master trainer and is certified by ACE as a health coach (HC), personal trainer (CPT), group fitness instructor (GFI), and cancer exercise specialist. She holds numerous certifications through Athletics and Fitness Association of America (AFAA). The recipient of the 2003 IDEA International Fitness Instructor of the Year award, she was inducted into the United States–based National Fitness Hall of Fame in 2007.

Originally from Australia, Roberts moved to the United States in 1990 to pursue her passion—fitness! She quickly became one of the most in demand private trainers in Los Angeles and garnered a celebrity clientele that included Cher, Kirstie Alley, Jennifer Grey, Jennifer Jason Leigh, Russell Crowe, and Faye Dunaway, and her step classes attracted stars such as Julia Roberts, Annette Bening, and Jennifer Beals.

Roberts is also a successful author and has been featured in *Shape, Elle, Health, Fitness, Self, Ms Fitness, American Fitness, Allure,* and many international publications. She has designed, choreographed, and starred in over 80 fitness videos and DVDs, including the award-winning video *Cher Fitness: A New Attitude.*

As CEO and owner of Keli's Real Fitness Inc., Roberts trains a variety of clients, including pregnant women, new mothers, and senior citizens. She works with clients with multiple sclerosis, cancer, and cardiac issues as well as those who have been in physical therapy. She teaches group fitness classes at Equinox in Pasadena and Glendale, and at Breakthru Fitness in Pasadena.

She conducts continuing education seminars, workshops, and master classes worldwide. She is a faculty member for SCW Fitness Education, a senior master trainer for Schwinn, and a BOSU elite developmental team member.

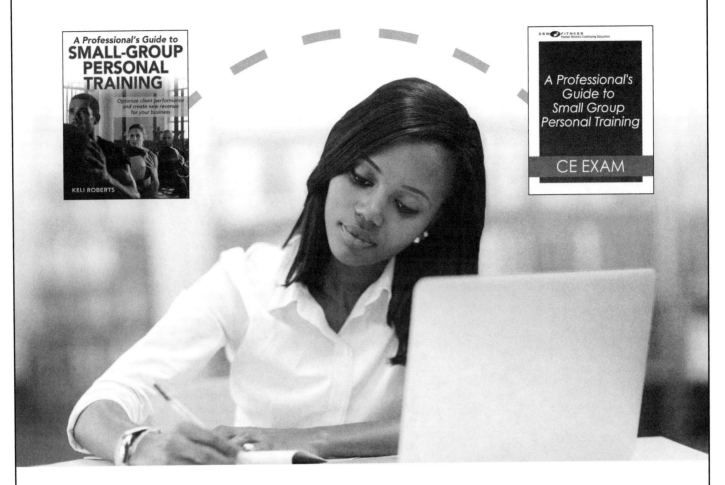
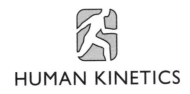